JUN 2 1 2019

P9-CKE-826

NAPA COUNTY LIBRARY
580 COOMBS STREET
NAPA, CA 94559

Praise for Expecting Mindfully

"As the mom of a 2-year-old with another on the way, this book has helped me be present and manage the stresses and craziness of this hectic time. I now have the tools to help me slow down when I feel worn out or overwhelmed by it all, and can react in a mindful, deliberate manner. The book has also helped me see the beauty in the messy moments. I can savor this stage instead of allowing sleep deprivation to let my mind drift on autopilot."

—Erin C., North Wales, Pennsylvania

"There are so many books for expecting and new mothers, but few so gently and wisely share evidence-based methods to quiet our busy minds and calm our distress. Take your time to work through this book and give yourself the gifts that it offers. You will find enduring tools to carry you through all the ups and downs of parenthood."

—Wendy N. Davis, PhD, Executive Director,
Postpartum Support International

"The emotional habits you bring to pregnancy and giving birth—such as believing you need to be a 'perfect' mother—can get in the way of taking care of yourself. *Expecting Mindfully* prepares you for the mental and emotional challenges that accompany having a baby, so you can get your mind ready, not just the baby's room! This book offers a powerful mix of mindfulness, cognitive therapy, and practical wisdom that will help you during and after pregnancy—and all through life."

—Tara Bennett-Goleman, MA, author of Emotional Alchemy,
and Daniel Goleman, PhD, author of Emotional Intelligence

"Women often don't receive the help they need for the very common feelings of depression, anxiety, and stress during pregnancy. The program in this book can help you stay emotionally well at this exciting but sometimes difficult time. Using two of the most well-established techniques in therapy today could benefit all pregnant women!"

—Vivette Glover, PhD, Professor of Perinatal Psychobiology,
Imperial College London, United Kingdom

"The writing style makes you feel like you are having a heartfelt conversation with the authors, as well as a supportive group of other expecting and new mothers. I only wish I'd had this book when I was first expecting!"

—Blakie S., Guelph, Ontario, Canada

"This book is an absolute gem. It pulls back the curtain on your mental health needs as an expectant or new mother and provides proven tools to address them. Drs. Dimidjian and Goodman's unique blend of clinical wisdom and research, coupled with Sharon Salzberg's guided meditations, engages both your heart and mind in this vital work."

—Zindel Segal, PhD, coauthor of The Mindful Way
through Depression

"Pregnancy was daunting for me. I was overwhelmed and anxious about my ever-growing body, the baby's health, and my new role as a mother. This compassionate workbook helped me find solid ground in tempestuous seas. I will be forever grateful to Drs. Dimidjian and Goodman for helping me enjoy my pregnancy and equipping me with the tools to be a mindful parent."

—*Christie-Anne L., Boulder, Colorado*

"This user-friendly book will help you avoid the heartache of postpartum depression by creating your own early warning system. I wish this resource had been available when I was having my children."

—*Nanette Santoro, MD, Professor of Obstetrics and Gynecology, University of Colorado*

"This book is an extraordinary achievement. All the activities are described in language that is easily understood. The authors convey warmth, sensitivity, and authentic concern for all women who are adapting to parenthood—especially those whose worries are preoccupying or who are feeling demoralized or pessimistic. There is practical guidance about how to integrate the program into a busy daily life, and many opportunities to shape it for individual circumstances."

—*Jane Fisher, AO, PhD, FCCLP, FCHP, clinical psychologist; Professor of Women's Health and Global Health, Monash University, Australia*

"As a father-to-be, this book has helped me understand my wife's feelings during her pregnancy, and also taught me some skills that I will be able to bring forward in our new life together as a family. The authors do an excellent job of walking you through the exercises in a logical manner while leaving lots of room to let your experience be your guide."

—*Michael B., Burnaby, British Columbia, Canada*

EXPECTING MINDFULLY

Expecting Mindfully

Nourish Your
Emotional Well-Being
and Prevent Depression
during Pregnancy and Postpartum ·

Sona Dimidjian, PhD
Sherryl H. Goodman, PhD

Audio meditations by Sharon Salzberg
Foreword by Samantha Meltzer-Brody

The Guilford Press
New York   London

Copyright © 2019 The Guilford Press
A Division of Guilford Publications, Inc.
370 Seventh Avenue, Suite 1200, New York, NY 10001
www.guilford.com

All rights reserved

The information in this volume is not intended as a substitute for consultation with healthcare professionals. Each individual's health concerns should be evaluated by a qualified professional.

Purchasers of this book have permission to copy forms, where indicated by footnotes, for personal use or use with clients. These forms may be copied from the book or accessed directly from the publisher's website, but may not be stored on or distributed from intranet sites, Internet sites, or file-sharing sites, or made available for resale. No other part of this book may be reproduced, translated, stored in a retrieval system, or transmitted, in any form or by any means, electronic, mechanical, photocopying, microfilming, recording, or otherwise, without written permission from the publisher.

See page 212 for terms of use for audio files.

Printed in the United States of America

This book is printed on acid-free paper.

Last digit is print number: 9   8   7   6   5   4   3   2   1

The following copyright holders have generously given permission to reprint material from copyrighted works:

From "Cognitive Self-Statements in Depression: Development of an Automatic Thoughts Questionnaire," by Steven D. Hollon, in *Cognitive Therapy and Research,* Vol. 4, Issue 4, pages 388–389. Copyright © 1980 Springer. Reprinted by permission of Springer.

From "The Guest House," by Jelaluddin Rumi (Coleman Barks, trans.). Copyright by Coleman Barks. Reprinted by permission of Coleman Barks.

Library of Congress Cataloging-in-Publication Data is available from the publisher.

ISBN 978-1-4625-2902-5 (paperback) — ISBN 978-1-4625-3247-6 (hardcover)

Illustrations by Erin Cantwell

Contents

Foreword   vii

Acknowledgments   ix

Our Journey Together   1

Getting Started   11

CLASS 1
Mindfulness Begins with the Everyday   21

CLASS 2
Body, Mind, and Breath   39

CLASS 3
Rhythms of Motherhood   61

CLASS 4
Opening to Difficulty and Uncertainty   85

CLASS 5
Thoughts Are Not Facts   113

CLASS 6
How Can I Best Take Care of Myself?   133

CLASS 7
Expanding Your Circle of Care   155

CLASS 8
Looking to the Future   179

Resources   201

Index   205

About the Authors   211

List of Audio and Video Tracks   212

Purchasers of this book can download select practical tools as well as audio and video files at *www.guilford.com/dimidjian-materials* for personal use or use with clients (see copyright page for details).

Foreword

Expecting Mindfully provides incredibly helpful tools and skills for women who are expecting or postpartum. This wonderful book is easy to read and offers highly practical and valuable information that all new mothers need. Drs. Sona Dimidjian and Sherryl Goodman, experts with decades of experience in the fields of perinatal mood disorders and parenting, bring mindfulness-based cognitive therapy directly to pregnant and postpartum women. With the evidence-based therapy described here, women can enjoy optimal overall health and well-being during the amazing transition to motherhood.

The perinatal period is a vulnerable time for women and their families. Even under the best circumstances, the transition to motherhood is challenging. Women struggle with unrealistic expectations about motherhood that can cause significant anxiety and mood symptoms. And women who have a history of depression frequently worry about relapse, even more so during pregnancy and the postpartum period. Furthermore, it can be difficult for women to find the time to engage in the self-care needed to maintain their well-being during this time. Given that women in many places lack access to specialized perinatal mental health providers, this book is a treasure chest of knowledge that makes a unique program available to all women who read and practice the skills presented here. The accompanying mindfulness meditation guides on audio and yoga instruction on video are especially helpful and well done.

This beautifully written book is one that all new mothers will want to read and is a welcome addition to the body of work available to perinatal women. Expecting Mindfully provides the tools women need to mindfully embrace the inherent chaos of motherhood. Moreover, it allows for the critical development and enhancement of new skills that will empower women to manage the normal demands and challenges that come with motherhood and beyond.

SAMANTHA MELTZER-BRODY, MD, MPH
The University of North Carolina at Chapel Hill

Acknowledgments

This work would not be possible without the collaboration and generous contributions of many people. First and foremost, we express our deep thanks to Zindel Segal and the gift that he, Mark Williams, and John Teasdale offered by creating the mindfulness-based cognitive therapy program. We have benefited greatly from their knowledge, expertise, writing, research, friendship, and collaboration. We hope that our adaptation of their work to benefit pregnant and early parenting women and their families does justice to their decades of work and innovation.

We also acknowledge funding by the National Institute of Mental Health (R34MH083866), which has allowed us to pursue this work with care and rigor. We want to thank all the study team members who contributed to our years of research with pregnant and postpartum moms—the basis for this book—including our key collaborators at the Institute for Health Research at Kaiser Permanente, Arne Beck and Jennifer Boggs, and, at West Chester University, Bob Gallop. Our appreciation goes to the prenatal care and mental health providers at Kaiser Permanente Colorado and Georgia who helped us connect with mothers who had the potential to benefit from this work: Amy Brooks-DeWeese, Deborah Hoerter, Thomas B. Landry, Fonda Mitchell, Carolee Nimmer, Robbin Ryan, and Joanne Whalen. We also express deep gratitude to all of the wonderful research team members at the University of Colorado and Emory University who supported the implementation of our research, including Abigail Lindemann, Abigail Lockhart, Allen Mallory, Courtney Timms, and Amanda Whittaker.

Our graduate students at the University of Colorado Boulder and Emory University have also been critical members of our research teams, and many of them carry forward a dedication to supporting pregnant and postpartum women and families in their own ongoing work. We acknowledge the amazing efforts of Jennifer Felder and Christina Metcalf, who were graduate students at the University of Colorado Boulder, and Amanda Brown Evans, who was at Emory University. Debra Boeldt, Christopher Hawkey, and Courtney Stevens, who were graduate students at the University of Colorado, and Cara Lusby, Meaghan McCallum, and Matthew Rouse, who were graduate students at Emory University, also played a critical role in conducting research evaluations with the moms who participated in the studies.

We would like to express special appreciation for the incredible wisdom and heartfulness of the contemplative teachers who contributed to this book: Sharon Salzberg, who collaborated on the writing and recording of the meditation instructions; Nancy Bardacke, who contributed consultation and the "Being with Baby" meditation practice; and De West, who recorded the yoga practices. We also express our gratitude to Kitty Moore and Chris Benton at The Guilford Press for their talented support and enthusiasm throughout the process of writing and completing this book.

I (Sona) express deep appreciation to all of my mentors and collaborators, who have guided me and enriched this work with wisdom and compassion. I also express my love and gratitude to the person who has been my most influential teacher about motherhood and mindfulness—my daughter, Serena. Her joyful presence reminds me every day that it is a blessing and responsibility to do this work. Finally, I thank the University of Colorado Boulder for being a place where the science and practice of mindfulness and wellness could take root and grow.

I (Sherryl) also offer appreciation to the teachers who encouraged and inspired me, including John MacKinnon, Don Meichenbaum, and Dick Steffy. This work rests on a foundation of warmth, support, and accumulated wisdom gathered from lifelong experiences with my parents, Bernard and Jeannette Goodman; my husband, Richard Snyder; and my sons, Josh and Seth Snyder; and additional treasured experiences with my daughters-in-law, Missy and Danielle, and granddaughter, Chloe.

Finally, our steadfast dedication to all women who struggle with depression in the context of parenting is an ever-present source of motivation to continue this work.

Our Journey Together

Sara* was no stranger to depression. Her mom had been depressed on and off when she was a child, and she had recently watched her youngest sister struggle under the weight of postpartum depression. She saw the heaviness that her sister carried with her every day, the struggle to connect with the experiences she had anticipated would bring her joy, the utter absence of motivation to do the daily tasks that were once routine for her, and the self-doubts about her ability to be a good mother that plagued her. Sara had been her sister's main support, finding information for her online about depression and insisting that they go to her 6-week obstetrics appointment together to talk with her doctor and get help. Sara also remembered what it felt like to be depressed herself, as she had struggled as a teenager and again after starting a demanding job with a very unpredictable schedule. She didn't want her sister to experience any of that while caring for her nephew.

When, shortly after helping her sister, Sara discovered that she was pregnant, she was filled with delight—and worry. She always knew that she wanted to be a mom and she had been trying to get pregnant for some time. She imagined the ways in which she would feel the pleasures of cuddling with the baby, the joys of the first smiles, the satisfaction of feeding and caring for the baby. She felt so strongly about the kind of mother she wanted to be and how she wanted to parent her child. Alongside this excitement and commitment, though, a sense of fear and dread took root in her belly. She knew that she was at higher risk of experiencing depression during pregnancy and the postpartum than other women who didn't have personal or family histories of depression. She knew the ways in which depression among mothers is tough on kids from her own childhood. She didn't want that for her child. She knew the ways in which depression can be hard on moms from witnessing the ways her sister had struggled. She didn't want that for herself. Being a new mother was hard enough without adding the weight of depression.

---

*All of the case examples, quotes, and vignettes are based on composites of women with whom we have worked or have been altered to disguise individual identities.

As Sara signed up for her birth classes and shopped for cribs and strollers, she reflected on how much our world focuses on preparing for the birth and the baby and how little focus there is on supporting pregnant women and new moms. People asked her all the time about the pregnancy; about her plans for the birth; about her ideas regarding names, and diapers, and all the other big and small decisions facing new parents. Few people, though, asked about how she was feeling or about steps she could be taking to support her own mental health during the ups and downs of pregnancy and the transition to the postpartum.

With all of the changes that motherhood would bring to her life, Sara knew that the period from pregnancy to the birth and the parenting of her infant would be challenging. Add depression, or vulnerability to depression, to that experience and the challenges can become overwhelming. Even now, the experience of excitement about what it would be like to raise her child and the sense of love and responsibility she felt for this new little being added stress to her life. Sara was committed to finding information and tools to support her own well-being. She knew that a big part of being the mother she dreamed of being was learning to cope with her vulnerability to depression and problems like anxiety and stress that were often present as well.

This book is designed to help you and other women like Sara maintain a sense of well-being during this important phase of your life. It's based on a proven program using mindfulness and cognitive-behavioral therapy that has helped thousands of people. It's designed to teach you skills for preventing depression, easing anxiety, and minimizing stress, skills that you can use throughout the journey of pregnancy, the postpartum, and early parenting (and, in fact, for the rest of your life!).

What Is This Program?

The program that teaches skills of such value for pregnant women and moms is called mindfulness-based cognitive therapy (MBCT), and our work has focused on adapting it specifically for women during pregnancy, postpartum, and early parenting. This book guides you through each step of the program, including the eight classes and all of the practices that you can do in your daily life. MBCT was created by Zindel Segal, Mark Williams, and John Teasdale, a team of psychologists from Canada and England. MBCT combines the practice of mindfulness with the strategies of cognitive-behavioral therapy in ways that are focused specifically on coping skillfully with challenges to prevent depression. If you haven't heard of cognitive-behavioral therapy or are not quite sure what it involves, it is one of the best-studied therapies, with strong evidence that it is helpful for treating depression and other problems. It teaches people how to change their ways of thinking and acting, which help improve problems like depression and anxiety. What does mindfulness add? As Segal, Williams, and Teasdale define it in *The Mindful Way Workbook,* "Mindfulness means being able to bring direct, open-hearted awareness to what you are doing while you are doing it: being able to tune in to what's going on in your mind and body, and in the outside world, moment by moment" (p. 5).

MBCT has been studied in many countries around the world, and nearly two decades of research demonstrate that thousands of women and men have benefited from the program. MBCT has helped them reduce the severity of depression, prevent relapses of depression, recognize emotional and cognitive reactions to stressful events, and live with greater wellness. In fact, one study pooled data from many other studies, which is a very strong test of effectiveness, and found that MBCT was as effective as staying on antidepressant medication in preventing relapses.

How Can This Program Help Women during Pregnancy, Postpartum, and Early Parenting?

We have adapted MBCT so that it retains the heart of the original program but is informed by 10 years of work we've done with pregnant, postpartum, and early parenting women to find out how MBCT could help specifically during this important and challenging time. What we learned helped us arrive at a program that supports expecting mindfully and staying well as a mom.

Our journey to this book began in 2004, around a conference table in Philadelphia at the Beck Institute for Cognitive Behavioral Therapy. We had both been invited to attend a year-long program as Beck Institute scholars. Participating in the program promised to provide a world of valuable learning about how to help people struggling with depression and related problems like anxiety and stress. Neither of us knew, however, that this great honor was going to change the course of our lives.

Two Researchers, One Goal

As a professor in the psychology department at Emory University in Atlanta, one of us, Sherryl, had studied moms and their babies in her lab for decades and had developed expertise in how depression affects mothers' parenting and their babies' development. Discoveries such as the fact that mothers with higher levels of depression symptoms are less accurate in identifying babies' positive emotions suggested that the negative bias associated with depression may extend to moms' experiences with their babies. By the time of the Beck Institute conference, Sherryl had mapped the territory of risk among women with histories of depression.

Sona's interest in MBCT started as a fascination during high school with meditation and its potential to help with depression. When the first major study on the effectiveness of MBCT was published, Sona became intrigued by the program. During graduate school in Seattle, she started working with a psychologist in Seattle to deliver the MBCT program to adults who had histories of depression. A memorable participant in one of the early groups was a mom with a toddler who described enthusiastically how she did the practices at home with her little one beside her. During the final class, she told Sona how the program had helped her develop skills that she believed would keep her well for years to come and that supported her now in being the mom she had always wanted to be. Walking out the door, she mentioned in passing, "I only wish I had learned this while I was pregnant; it would have saved us all a lot of suffering in those early months of the postpartum."

This idea lingered in Sona's memory and, combined with Sherryl's interests and experience, became the seeds of the program in this book. For Sherryl, focusing on helping women alter the risks that came with a vulnerability to depression seemed like a natural next step. For Sona, finding a like-minded scientist whose passionate interest converged with hers felt like the best possible stroke of luck. When we realized that we were at an important transition in our own experiences of motherhood—Sona having left her 3-year-old daughter for the first time to attend the conference and Sherryl having just sent her son off to college—the collaboration seemed like it was meant to be.

Together, following the meeting at the Beck Institute, we applied for and received a grant from the National Institute of Mental Health to conduct a study adapting MBCT for women during pregnancy. We spent years working with pregnant women to refine the MBCT program to be as supportive as possible for women during pregnancy and the postpartum. We taught the MBCT course, in Colorado and Georgia, and we learned by reflecting together, with the women in the classes, with our graduate students (who fell in love with this work as much as we had), and with our other collaborators. We learned along the way from other experts in the field, including Nancy Bardacke, who contributed practices from her work on childbirth and parenting. We also had the great fortune to work closely with Sharon Salzberg, a bestselling author, much loved teacher of mindfulness meditation, and now our dear friend. Sharon recorded all of the practice guides we used in our studies, and it is her voice you will hear guiding you in the practices that accompany this book (see page 212 for more information).

In our first published study, we enrolled 49 pregnant women, and all of them received the MBCT classes, which we worked to customize for their experiences and needs during pregnancy and the postpartum. All had experienced depression in the past, and none were seriously depressed when they enrolled. We found that women liked the classes and did the home practices we recommended to support their learning. The women also experienced a significant reduction in their depressive symptoms over time, which is important because even mild symptoms of depression can be hard on moms and babies during pregnancy and the postpartum period.

In our second published study, we enrolled 86 women, half of whom received the MBCT classes that we had customized for women during pregnancy, and the other half received usual care in the Kaiser Permanente system. Only 18% of the women who received the MBCT classes experienced a relapse of depression through 6 months postpartum, compared with 50% of women who received usual care. The women who were protected from the return of depression learned and practiced the very same skills and lessons that we share with you in this book.

Is This Book for Me?

The program in this book is for you if:

- You're pregnant, postpartum, or in early motherhood and want to maintain the best possible overall health and well-being.

- You're vulnerable to depression, having been depressed at other times in your life or because you have other risk factors for depression (see the box below to learn about risk factors for depression during pregnancy, postpartum, and early parenting).

- You're concerned about the effects of feeling "down," stressed, or anxious on your parenting and the well-being of your baby.

- You're looking for ways to stay well that pose the least risk for your baby and your own physical health.

You can use this workbook if you're experiencing residual symptoms of depression—but we do not recommend this program as a first response to an acute episode of depression (see

---

What Are Some Risk Factors for Depression during Pregnancy, Postpartum, and Early Parenting?

- Personal history of depression
- Personal history of anxiety
- History of depression in your family
- Recent stressful life events
- Low social supports
- Stress in your marriage or partnership
- Financial stress
- Low self-esteem
- Complications during labor and delivery
- Stress with your baby

the box below to learn what these terms mean). You can benefit from this book even if you don't use words like "depression" to describe your experience but find yourself saying often that you are "overwhelmed" or "stressed" or having a "hard time," even if only to yourself, or have said that about yourself in the past. For many women, being depressed, anxious, or stressed comes with a vulnerability to self-criticism; this book can help there too—along with helping you protect yourself from being criticized as a mother by others.

Do you need to be familiar with mindfulness meditation or cognitive-behavioral therapy to get the most out of the book? Not at all. As noted above, MBCT helps people change their

---

What Is Acute Depression?

To determine if changes in how a woman is feeling indicate depression, mental health professionals pay attention to specific symptoms of depression and to the frequency and duration of these symptoms and the degree to which the symptoms get in the way of her usual functioning. The symptoms include:

- Little interest or pleasure in doing things
- Feeling down, depressed, or hopeless
- Trouble falling or staying asleep, or sleeping too much
- Feeling tired or having little energy
- Poor appetite or overeating
- Feeling bad about yourself—or that you are a failure or have let yourself or your family down
- Trouble concentrating on things, such as reading the newspaper or watching TV
- Moving or speaking so slowly that other people could have noticed. Or the opposite—being so fidgety or restless that you have been moving around a lot more than usual
- Thoughts that you would be better off dead, or of hurting yourself in some way

Acute depression, or "an episode of major depression," refers to a period of at least 2 weeks during which at least five of these symptoms (of which one must be the first or second) are present for most of the day, nearly every day, and get in the way of a woman's ability to carry out normal daily activities. If this is the case for you, we recommend that you reach out to a mental health professional to talk about treatment options. Come back to this program at another time to learn skills that will help you maintain your recovery and stay well over time.

relationship with their thoughts and emotions so that the ways they respond to challenges are less likely to lead to anxiety and depression, especially given the new challenges of being pregnant or parenting an infant. You'll become familiar with all of this information in the eight classes that follow.

Perhaps more than anything else, this book is for you if you want to take an active role in defining what wellness means to you and how you choose to stay well during pregnancy and the postpartum.

How Can This Program Help Me?

The skills of mindfulness and cognitive-behavioral therapy are always available. They don't require special equipment or even additional time. We know that this is essential for women during pregnancy and the postpartum, who have so many demands on their time. At any time, you can shift your attention to present-moment experience—and this shift can help you stay well. It's a simple shift, but one that requires practice. Learning the skills of this program will help you step out of old patterns that place you at risk for depression, anxiety, and stress and step into new patterns that nourish your well-being and your relationship with your baby and other important people in your life, such as your partner, friends, or older children.

We will guide you through eight classes, each of which invite you to learn in two ways: through reading and through practice. The reading will provide you with important information about depression, anxiety, and stress and the ways in which this program can help you stay well. Because it is not possible to learn through reading alone, each class also will invite you to learn from your experience. In this way, this class is different from many other prenatal and postpartum classes you might take. As one mother said: "I was expecting it to be kind of like any other class you go to while you are pregnant; I mean you go to breastfeeding class and CPR class. But this was totally different. Those other classes are really about learning information. This was so much more than that. The practices that I learned and paying attention to how I felt and what I noticed and how that awareness helps me stay well, that was the heart of the class. It was really learning from my experience and paying attention."

We begin the eight classes with a focus on concrete and accessible experiences, like what we feel moment to moment in the body while eating, lying down, breathing, and walking. Over time, we move to practices that focus more on emotions and thoughts, including ones that are difficult. Moving along with this sequence helps to build the skill of mindfulness in daily routine ways, before addressing the difficult moments in your life. It's like lifting weights, building your strength and skill with 5-pound weights before you take on the 25-pound ones.

Countering Isolation with Circles of Connection

Having a baby and the experience of depression can be isolating for many women. And being depressed or anxious can be stressful for other people in your life. Family and friends, who may have been supportive at first, can become confused and distant over time. Conversely, they may not understand the ways that things are changing for you and that it is not possible for you to do all the same things to support them that you were doing before you became pregnant or had a new baby. Building support for yourself and keeping a balance between how much you give and how much you receive is an essential part of staying well. This workbook will guide you in many ways in creating circles of connection that support you.

With the importance of connections in mind, first, we want you to know that you will not be learning alone. In each class, you will be learning from the experiences of other women as reflected in their comments about the practices and program. You will see sections in each chapter labeled "circle of mothers," and these sections give voice to the experiences of other women, each of whom struggled with depression and problems like stress, anxiety, and feeling overwhelmed. Each of them also wanted the best for her baby and her experience of motherhood. These mothers will share with you the ways in which the practices of mindfulness have been important. You will have opportunities to reflect on your own experiences and add your voice to theirs.

Second, we will guide you in expanding the circles of support in your everyday life. As part of getting started, we will invite you to choose a support person to travel with you on this journey to well-being. This support person can be your husband, partner, sister, mother, other relative, or friend. Another option, if you have a psychotherapist or counselor, is to suggest that you work through these classes with his or her support. Other women might choose to invite a group of friends to complete this workbook together. Know, though, that you need only one person as a support as you get started.

The main role of the support person is to help you keep your commitment to reading the workbook chapters and doing the daily practices. When you encounter barriers to practice, your support person can remind you of your motivation to do the classes or brainstorm with you about how to get help with other work, child care, or household tasks so that you have time to do the daily practices. Staying connected with your support person is intended to help you stay connected to this program. You may find that keeping the people who are close to you involved in what you are learning can be helpful for them as well as for you.

Third, we will teach you specific skills for asking others for help and saying no to requests that are not in the best interest of your well-being. As one mother who completed this program explained: "The mindfulness practices and all the skills I've learned in this program have helped me to ask for help. I am able to tell people and not be afraid to be honest with them about how I'm feeling and when I'm having a hard time. For many years, I always put a really positive façade out there and wouldn't let people know that I was struggling. It left me really alone and overwhelmed. Through this program, I've reached out to and engaged my support system, which I didn't do in the past. If I am not doing well I tell them, and if I am doing well I tell them. It's made a big difference in my life. And I think it helps my family too, because they're less worried and they now know what they can do to help me."

Your Safety

We want to support your emotional safety as you think about doing this program. As mentioned above, if you are experiencing an acute episode of depression, this is not the optimal time to do this program. Many effective treatments for depression exist, and we have included information in the Resources section at the back of the book to guide you in finding an effective treatment in your area. Depression is treatable. We encourage you to connect with a professional mental health provider. After your depression is treated, you may want to return to this book to learn practices and skills to help you prevent future episodes of depression. For now, though, we want you to get the treatment help that you and your baby need.

We also want to help support your physical safety. Before you begin any physical activity during pregnancy, including the yoga and walking practices that we integrate into this program, we recommend that you consult with your health care provider. It is important to talk with your provider about whether you have any health conditions that would limit your participation in the yoga or any other practices in this program. Your health care professional can offer advice about what kind of physical activity is best for you. Also, please read the guidelines regarding physical activity during pregnancy published by the American College of Obstetrics and Gynecology (*www.acog.org/Patients/FAQs/Exercise-During-Pregnancy*); if you notice any warning signs, please stop your activity and contact your health care provider. If you have the support of your health care provider to do the movement practices, you can integrate the practices that we include in Class 3. If you do not have approval to do the movement practices, it is absolutely fine to skip those parts of the program and focus on the other practices.

The Value of Your Time

When we were writing this workbook, we shared drafts of the classes with pregnant women and new moms whom we know had struggled with depression. The chapters you will be reading integrate their wisdom as well as that of the women we taught in person. One message we heard loud and clear from their feedback was this: caution moms that it takes time to learn these skills and that learning is not always easy. You will be asked to dedicate time each day. Other moms have told us that on some days that feels all but impossible. Don't be surprised if this is true for you. In the eight classes, we offer suggestions for how to work with this challenge of time. For now, we want to alert you that you are in good company if you struggle with limited time and fatigue, and it's possible to make your way through any rough patches with the guidance and support that we and the circle of mothers provide.

And Now . . .

We encourage you to read the "Getting Started" chapter to begin this journey with us. The practical tips and emotional guidance offered provide an essential foundation for your learning for the eight classes that follow.

Getting Started

*I believe we learn by practice. Whether it means to learn to
dance by practicing dancing or to learn by practicing living,
the principles are the same.*

—Martha Graham

All journeys are made easier by spending some time preparing. In this chapter, we share some of the practicalities of this course, such as scheduling, timing, and supplies. We also help you know what to expect from each class and the practices you will be invited to do each day between classes. Finally, because this is a journey that will be made easier by engaging the support of others, we explore ways to connect with your own inner conviction and with others in your life.

Practical Preparations for the Journey

We encourage you to consider an 8-week structure for using this book, taking one day of the week to read one chapter and spending the other days of the week doing the daily practices, as the women in our research did. Can you identify an 8-week period on your calendar that will allow you to fully commit to this program, including the daily practice? Because the classes build progressively over time, it's best to do the classes in order.

At the same time, as you will learn, a key emphasis of this program is paying attention to how you feel and how to best support your well-being. So, if you find that stretching out the program, say, to complete one chapter over 2 or 3 weeks is helpful, you might experiment with that approach. As one mom who completed this workbook reflected: "I think the real benefit is to be able to do the program at one's own pace. Unlike most therapy or other programs like this, the workbook doesn't require one to take up extensive amounts of time and money to get help, and you can do it when and how it works for you."

We also recommend that you:

- *Find a quiet place to read each chapter.* It's important that the place be comfortable and as free from distraction as possible.

- *Identify a specific day of the week to read each new chapter.* You can anticipate that it will take about an hour to two to read and complete the practices as you work your way through each chapter for the first time. You might consider adding this time to your calendar right now.

In whatever ways you use this workbook, please give yourself permission to use your own experience as a guide—paying attention to when it's helpful to take a little more time with a chapter and when it's helpful to move on, as well as the specific locations and times of day during which you read and practice with the chapters. Ultimately, what matters is making your way through the workbook.

You'll also need some equipment that's best to line up in advance:

- A tablet, smart phone, computer, or other device to access the audio and video recordings of the guided practices that are available through online downloads (p. 212)

- A chair or cushions for your meditation practice, ideally both, so you can choose to sit on a chair or on the floor as your preference changes across pregnancy and the postpartum (Class 3 provides instructions.)

- A yoga mat if you have approval from your health care professional to do the yoga practice. (Plan to use either the guided yoga practice and videos in this book or another option for prenatal and postpartum yoga, available at many local yoga studios, gyms, health facilities, and online.)

What to Expect from Each Class and the Daily Practices

Each class follows a similar structure:

Three Lessons

Each chapter contains three lessons to guide your learning. In these core lessons, we offer all we have learned from our work over the years with pregnant and postpartum women and the best available knowledge about how to prevent depression and support well-being. These lessons are designed to help you support yourself and your family through these important life transitions.

Practice and Reflection

Each chapter provides instructions for practices to do while reading, which are indicated with the symbol of a heart (shown at right), and reflection questions to support you in learning from the most powerful teacher: your own experience. Developing the skill of mindfulness is much like growing a plant; attending with care each day allows the flower to blossom fully over time.

Each reflection opportunity is an invitation to be curious about your own experience. There are no right or wrong answers. Generally, the reflection questions follow a similar structure that you can envision as a set of concentric circles; see the figure below:

- *The "innermost" circle.* We always begin with asking you to reflect on what you noticed about your direct experience in the practice: what you saw, felt, heard, and so forth. We encourage you to practice staying close to the direct experience that you just had. When we reflect on practices, it's common to go past the immediate experience and relate it to something else. For example, instead of reflecting on the sweet taste of a strawberry, one might move automatically to telling the story of the wonderful strawberries you ate last summer. Direct experiences, like tasting, are often missed when we focus on stories *about* the experience rather than the experience itself. Short and simple responses—sweet, salty, rough, pungent, and so forth—often help keep you close to the experience when answering the first set of reflection questions.

- *The "middle" circle.* Here we expand to inquire about how this mindful experience differed from your usual mode. For example, you might reflect on how eating a

Reflections on Practice: Three Levels

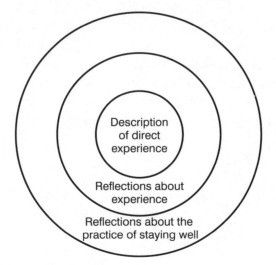

Description
of direct
experience

Reflections about
experience

Reflections about the
practice of staying well

strawberry mindfully is quite different from your typical eating habits, such as not noticing the sensations of tasting when eating while talking, driving, or rushing to the next activity.

- *The "outer" circle.* Finally, we invite you to reflect on the ways in which the practice is relevant to your staying well over time, particularly during the important time of pregnancy and postpartum. For staying well, we want you to focus on what that means for you. For many, it means preventing depression's return or reducing the lingering symptoms of depression. For others, it also means reducing anxiety. For others still, it means specific actions that are linked to depression and anxiety risk and that are worthy in their own right, like eating healthfully or getting adequate sleep. At the end of this chapter, we will ask you to describe what "staying well" means for you. This will be an important anchor for your reflections as you complete the practices in each chapter.

Circle of Mothers

Each practice and reflection section includes a "circle of mothers" that offers quotes from other women who are working to learn the same skills as you and to integrate them into their daily lives while pregnant and parenting. These are intended to stand in for the group in an in-person version of the program—picture yourself sitting in a welcoming, supportive circle of other women who share similar struggles and hopes for themselves and their children.

These women comment on their experiences of learning the practices, including what came easily and what was more challenging. They also comment on how they applied these skills to daily life over time, learning to respond more skillfully to various aspects of pregnancy, postpartum, and the shift into parenting. The circle of mothers speaks to the experience of learning the practices and skills and the impact, over time, on their day-to-day lives.

Following the circle of mothers, we include some guidance and recommendations about how to work with challenges and how to integrate the core skills in your daily life. These suggestions also represent the collective wisdom of many moms who have traveled along the same road to wellness. We encourage you to return to the experiences of the circle of mothers if you find yourself feeling discouraged, confused, or overwhelmed as you work through the lessons. Instead of giving up, please come back and lean on the experiences of other women who have traveled the same journey on which you are embarking.

Daily Practice and Journal

Invitations and instructions for daily practice assignments and a daily Practice Journal are included in each class to help you make the most of this program. You will find each of the practices highlighted with the symbol of a flower (shown at right) at the end of each lesson and summarized at the end of each chapter.

Each daily mindfulness practice is supported with an audio track that was recorded by an expert mindfulness teacher, Sharon Salzberg, or a video track (see page 212 for more information). The first time you do each practice, we recommend that you listen to the audio or watch the video guidance. After that, you may choose to practice without the audio or video guidance or return to them occasionally.

We teach two categories of practice: informal and formal. Each is important and supports the other.

- *Informal Practice*: Informal practices support you in weaving the skills of mindfulness into the everyday moments of your life. Every moment of your day provides an opportunity for mindfulness. As you are learning these skills, it is helpful to bring some structure and intention to practicing informally. For this reason, we include specific practices, such as mindful eating or washing dishes and mindfully being with your baby.

- *Formal Practice*: Formal practices invite you to let go of your to-do list and step out of the momentum and busyness of everyday life into this very moment in a way that is even more sustained than informal mindfulness practice. The formal practices invite you to set aside time for you, a time for turning inward, for nourishing and caring for yourself with your attention. It's helpful to identify a specific time of day to complete the formal daily practice assigned in each chapter to help you build the practice into your routine. You can anticipate that the formal daily practice will require about 25 minutes each day. It may be best for you to choose a specific time of day, so that it becomes part of your routine more easily. Also, it is helpful to find a quiet place to do the formal practices where you are unlikely to be interrupted and where you feel safe and comfortable.

- After each of your daily practice sessions, we recommend that you reflect on your experience and record some brief notes in your Practice Journal. If you find you want more space to record your thoughts, a blank form that you can use for any of the eight classes is available to download and print (see the box at the end of the table of contents for more information).

Connecting with a Support Person

Gathering support for your journey is a key part of getting started. We will focus in Class 6 on how to engage a support team in the broader process of staying well. Here we focus more narrowly on identifying a support person who can help you fully participate in the program and put into practice the skills you are learning to stay well and prevent depression. At the end of each chapter, you will find guidelines for connecting with this support person and reflecting on what you learned. (If you find you need more space for these reflections, feel free to download and print the blank form we offer; see the box at the end of the table of contents for more information.) In the next section, we suggest some ideas to guide you in choosing the best support person for your journey.

Inviting and Sustaining Support for the Journey

As for any new skill, it takes time and repetition to make the practice of mindfulness your own and part of your everyday routine. For moms and moms-to-be, it can be hard to create time for yourself to read the chapters of this workbook and do daily practice.

Sometimes it's helpful to think what might happen if you were told the following: "There is something you can do for a friend or for your child that is very valuable and that can keep her well. It will take only a few minutes each day. Would you be willing to do it?" You would probably say yes. In fact, you might not even think twice.

This program is a chance to give yourself the same kind of gift that you would readily give to others. It's easy to put off taking care of ourselves when the demands of caring for others are high, as they are during pregnancy or with a new baby. These demands make the gift of the daily practices in this program even more valuable.

To help you create and sustain the support that is helpful for this journey, we invite you to consider how to connect with and obtain the support of others in your life, especially one specific support person.

To help you identify a support person, take a moment to think of the people in your life. From your perspective, who are the important people in your life? Who are the people with whom you have a sense of connection? Write their names and their relationship to you (e.g., Sally/ sister) on the circles of connection shown on the facing page, with those who are closest to you, the people who are most important in your life, in the center circle.

Reflecting on your circles of connection, identify and note below the person you plan to ask to be your support person for this program and when you will ask this person to work with you in this crucial way:

_____

_____

_____

You might be tempted to skip this part of the program and assume that it's not so important or that you can find your support person later. *We strongly recommend otherwise!* Women who have participated in our program have shared with us repeatedly the conviction that engaging the support person early is a key part of doing the program and building the circles of care that they need to stay well over time. Here's what one mom told us about this part of the program: "Honestly, I don't know if I would have been as dedicated to the daily practices had I not made a plan with my support person starting at the outset. I actually found that it was important to have two check-ins with my support system each week. The first was after I read the chapter so I could tell him what I was committing to doing in the coming week. Usually that check-in was pretty brief. The second was after completing a week's worth of practices, and those sometimes were longer conversations that really helped me reflect on what I was learning. Doing both of those check-ins helped me stay on track in a way that would have been really hard to do without that support."

If it's helpful, please reflect on this list of possible "talking points" when reaching out to your support person:

- I am starting a program that is designed to help me stay well during pregnancy and postpartum because I am vulnerable to depression/anxiety/stress.

- I want to do this program because (*elaborate on your goals and vision, such as being the best mom you can be for yourself, your baby, and your family, based on your reflection on pages 18–19*):

- This program asks that I commit to working my way through a series of chapters with lessons and practices to do each day. There are eight chapters that build on each other in a systematic way over time.

My Circles of Connection

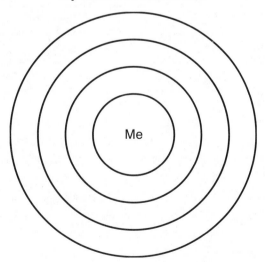

- I anticipate that it will require 1–2 hours to read the chapter each week and then 25–30 minutes per day to do the daily practices.

- I would like you to be my support person because (*elaborate here on why you selected this person and what this person means to you*).

- If you agree to be my support person, what I would ask of you is to talk with me after I complete each chapter, so that I can review with you what I am learning and explore any barriers to completing the program and how best to overcome them with your support. Some of the barriers that I anticipate may be challenging for me include (*elaborate here on potential barriers you have identified, based on your reflection on the facing page*).

- I would be very grateful if you would support me in this way. I think it will be very helpful to me, and you might learn useful information too!

Supporting Yourself

Given the presence of other demands in your life during pregnancy and parenting, it can be helpful as you are getting started to reflect on why *you* are making a commitment to doing this program and what you hope to learn. Take a few moments now to jot down your own personal reasons and how you hope to benefit.

What led you to start this journey? What are your hopes?

_____

_____

_____

_____

_____

_____

The heart of this program is developing the skills and practices to know yourself—how you are feeling, what you are thinking, what you want and don't want, and what will support you in living the life you value through your pregnancy, early parenting, and beyond. Sometimes it's tempting to take on others' ideas about how to live our lives. As we begin this journey, we invite you to reflect on what staying well means specifically for you. It's not about how someone else defines staying well but what will really serve you. This is important because it will be an anchor for you as you proceed through the eight classes. It's okay if you are unsure about what you value or want in your life or how you define staying well. Know that your understanding will become clearer and may change as you learn the skills in the eight classes. Consider this invitation right now as a time to jot down what comes to mind, knowing that you can add, revise, and build on these ideas over time.

With this in mind, what is your vision for staying well during pregnancy, postpartum, and beyond?

_____

_____

_____

_____

_____

_____

Now we invite you to pause for a moment and imagine what might get in the way of realizing your vision for staying well and giving yourself the gift of time to do this program and the daily practices that are a core part of our eight-class journey.

What barriers might you encounter on this path toward your vision of well-being?

_____

_____

_____

_____

_____

_____

If you struggle later with making the time for completing the workbook chapters and for practicing each day, you can refer back to these reflections—staying connected to the hopes that brought you to this journey, your vision of what staying well means and "looks like" for you.

As Mother Teresa said, "Yesterday is gone. Tomorrow has not yet come. We have only today. Let us begin."

We are excited to begin this journey with you.

CLASS 1

Mindfulness Begins with the Everyday

Better is silence. . . . Let me sit with bare things, this coffee cup, this knife, this fork, things in themselves, myself being myself.

—Virginia Woolf

This chapter focuses on three key lessons:

1. **We all have the ingredients necessary to learn mindfulness.** We invite you to begin the journey of mindfulness with everyday objects and activities.

2. **We all sometimes operate on autopilot, which has both benefits and costs.** We help you learn how to recognize autopilot in the context of daily life.

3. **You can learn to direct your attention intentionally rather than being pulled without awareness by autopilot.** We invite you to explore how the practice of the body scan can help you direct your attention.

Lesson 1. Mindfulness Is Always Available

How much is your attention focused on what you are doing right now, right here, in this very moment?

If you notice that your attention is elsewhere, or that it is here but only for a fleeting moment before being whisked away to some other distraction, demand, or desire, you are not alone.

Consider, for a moment, how much of your time is spent not paying full attention to what you are doing. How often do you notice that your attention gets pulled from one thing to another, perhaps thinking about what you need to do later today or replaying a conversation that happened yesterday? How often does a running commentary play in your mind alongside what you are doing, typically with a critical or pressured tone? "You'll never get this done." "This place is a mess!" "What were you thinking?!"

What would it feel like to be free of this running commentary and of getting pulled into the past or the future? It may seem unlikely (or even unimaginable), but it *is* possible to learn skills that offer this freedom. That is what the practice of mindfulness is all about. Not only is it possible, but you have everything you need to start learning right in your own kitchen.

People sometimes assume that mindfulness is some kind of complicated activity, perhaps thinking, "Other people can learn it, but it wouldn't work for me." In fact, you have the ingredients for the recipe of mindfulness already present in your everyday life. Learning mindfulness doesn't require trips to special stores or online orders. We will start with objects you can find in your refrigerator or on your cupboard shelves.

We invite you, now, to go into your kitchen and choose two small edible objects—raisins, nuts, pieces of fruit or candy, or whatever else is on hand. Once you have them, come back to your practice location and follow the instructions below; we suggest that you read the instructions and pause to practice after each paragraph.

As you are doing this, you may notice that thoughts pop into your mind: "Why am I spending so much time on a walnut?!" or "What does this have to do with staying well during pregnancy or taking care of my baby?!" At these moments when thoughts grab your attention, we invite you to notice, "There's a thought popping up," and then bring your attention back to the object. This may happen again and again, and each time we invite you to notice thinking and to bring your attention back. If your thoughts pull you far away, you can read the paragraph again if it's helpful to anchor you back in the practice.

Practice Now

Hold one object of food in the palm of your hand or between your finger and thumb and bring your attention to seeing the object as though you had never seen anything like it before. Look closely and carefully at the object, perhaps turning it over or rotating it to explore all of its sides. Explore seeing areas of light and shadow, color, shape. Let your eyes explore every part of it.

Now allow your focus on seeing the object to fade into the background of your awareness and bring your attention to the sensations of touching the object. You don't need to do anything differently, as you've been holding the object all along, but now focus your awareness on how it feels to touch the object. Notice texture—smooth, sharp, rough, sticky, dry. Perhaps roll the object between your fingers, exploring its texture.

Now bring your awareness to smelling the object. Hold the object just below your nostrils, noticing any scent as you inhale. Notice whatever is present in this moment—intense or mild scent or no scent at all. Allow yourself to explore the experience of smelling the object.

Now, allowing awareness of smelling to fade into the background, slowly place the object into your mouth, bringing your full awareness to the sensations of having the object in your mouth. Without chewing, notice the texture of the object on your tongue. Move the object around your mouth, perhaps also notice saliva forming in your mouth.

Now, when you are ready, bite into the object and notice any taste that it releases. Notice sensations of tasting, exploring what it feels like to taste the object with all of its flavors. You might even notice the urge to swallow when it arises and then notice the experience of swallowing.

Now we invite you to close your eyes and do the practice with the second object, moving your attention at your own pace from seeing to touching to smelling to tasting. If thoughts pull your attention away from the object, we invite you to notice "There's a thought popping into my mind" to bring your attention back to the object. When you have finished tasting the object, allow your eyes to open and reflect on your experiences.

Reflections on Practice

As we explained on page 7, you can't learn mindfulness and the ways in which it can help you stay well just by reading. It requires both direct experience and then reflecting on that experience. In reflecting on what you noticed, please remember that this is an opportunity to be curious about your experience. There are no right or wrong answers.

What sensations of seeing, touching, smelling, and tasting did you notice?

_____

_____

_____

_____

Circle of Mothers

"The surface of the walnut was so rough and hard."

"The candy was really shiny."

"I was really excited by the time we got to tasting, but the chocolate actually tasted kind of sharp."

"I didn't notice any smell when I had the raisin by my nostrils."

"I was thinking a lot about other stuff during a lot of the practice, but tasting was easier for me. The strawberry was really juicy and sweet."

"I was very distracted. I chose a raisin, and I noticed myself trying to define it, thinking 'This looks like a newborn baby's skin' and thinking about babies. I was going off in all these different directions, and it was hard to focus on my sensations."

How did the experiences of eating the object differ from your typical experience of eating?

_____

_____

_____

_____

_____

Circle of Mothers

"I usually eat my dinner in that whole time span, so this was totally different from how I normally eat. I'm usually eating while I'm at work or feeding the kids, so I don't really have the time to notice all the parts like I did just now. I don't really notice, as much as I love food, or cooking or preparing food, I don't usually take it all in. I think I miss a lot of the positives every day because I'm just not paying attention."

"This practice really showed me how my mind is in the past or future, not the present. I think it's exactly this same thing that makes me vulnerable to getting depressed. I don't even realize I'm doing it, but somehow I'm reviewing all the reasons that I'm screwing up at work or being a bad mom or whatever it is. Or I'm worrying about my kids' futures and how we are going to pay the bills. I'm not paying attention to the present like I did in this practice."

"It was really hard to slow down, because I have so much to do that if I don't feel like there's a purpose to something, it's hard. I feel like I have to be doing something all the time. I just wanted to get to the end."

As you reflect on your vision for staying well during pregnancy, postpartum, and beyond, described on page 19 how might this practice support you along the staying-well path?

_____

_____

_____

_____

_____

(**Circle of Mothers**)

"Staying well, for me, means having more peace of mind. I get it—with three kids under five and a full-time job, there won't be much peace in the house, but my mind just goes everywhere, all the time, and that brings me to the point of feeling overwhelmed on a daily basis. If you're overwhelmed with thoughts about whatever it is that you're trying to accomplish and then you just feel like you can't do any of it . . . , for me, that can contribute to a feeling of just hopelessness. It seems like when I am thinking too much, it could be really valuable to recognize that my thoughts are everywhere and learn how to rein them back in."

"I want to have less tension in my life. Here, I was like so relaxed that entire exercise. I just was very calm, and so I was noticing just by focusing on whatever it was at the moment—whether it was the touch, the seeing, the smell—I was, I was very relaxed. I think this practice might help."

"Focusing on the smells and tastes was really hard. I hardly focused on the candy at all, and when I noticed that I was distracted, I kept thinking that I was doing it wrong and that this is only the first class . . . how am I going to do eight classes if I can't even eat a piece of candy right!?"

A Recipe for Mindfulness. Through the practice of mindful eating, you may have realized how little of the time we are aware of experiences and how the practice provides a concrete way to shift attention. It also provides a direct experience of the fact that learning the skills of mindfulness doesn't require special equipment or even additional time. Mindfulness is always available. If you are like many during pregnancy and the postpartum, with demands on your energy and time, this is essential. That's where the daily practice comes in. Fortunately, all of the activities that one is busy doing every day also can provide an opportunity to practice mindfulness. The kitchen is a wonderful place to start your daily practice—with the routine, daily activities of eating, drinking, and cleaning. While doing any of these activities, you can shift your attention to the experience of simply being in the present moment—just as you did in eating just now—and this shift can help support you on the staying-well path. It's a simple shift, but one that requires practice.

Daily Practice for Lesson 1

As you've now practiced learning the skill of mindfulness with the edible objects from your kitchen, for the next 7 days, we invite you to practice bringing mindfulness to a daily activity.

- ◆ Listen to the "Introduction to Daily Activities" (Track 1) for an overview of the mindfulness of daily activities.

- ◆ Practice at least once a day with one of the daily activities: "Drinking Tea Meditation" (Track 2), "Eating Meditation" (Track 3), or "Washing Dishes Meditation" (Track 4). You may listen to the recordings for mindful drinking, eating, and washing dishes each time you practice or only the first few times and then explore bringing mindfulness to the activity on your own.

- ◆ In short and simple responses, record what you noticed in your Practice Journal at the end of this chapter. Focus on the sensations of seeing, touching, smelling, or tasting (e.g., "hot," "cool"). You also may notice and record where your mind was during the practice (e.g., "My mind wandered to worrying about the ultrasound").

Lesson 2. Expanding beyond the Kitchen: Noticing Autopilot

The practice of eating mindfully highlights the fact that many of us miss opportunities to be focused on our experience. We eat without being aware of the actual sensations of eating. This is autopilot. In our busy, everyday lives, we can sometimes go "on autopilot" for hours (or days!) without really being aware of it.

Autopilot certainly is useful at times. It can be very efficient, which is important when juggling the demands of pregnancy and a new baby. For example, autopilot can be helpful in the middle of the night when you need to change a diaper and prepare a bottle. But, when it's our only or main mode, autopilot comes with a cost. Autopilot may deprive us of fully experiencing the pleasurable moments of life. For example, we may be on autopilot going through the tasks of daily life—working, doing laundry, feeding and changing the baby—to the extent that we don't fully savor the moments when our babies make eye contact or smile or laugh.

If we've struggled with self-criticism and judgment or anxiety and worry, autopilot also may carry us into difficult territory without our awareness. All of a sudden, we're feeling down and don't know how we got there.

Doing Mode and Being Mode. For most mothers, much of daily life can be conducted on an autopilot "doing mode"—doing tasks, running errands, juggling responsibilities—with your awareness on getting to the next moment rather than fully experiencing the moment that you are in. In this way, "doing" can eclipse the moment-to-moment experience of "being."

Mindfulness practice—even just a few minutes every day—can offer the opportunity to notice how it feels to be in "doing mode" and to step into "being mode."

Mindfulness Is an Alternative to Autopilot. Practicing mindfulness—in concrete and direct ways, like eating with awareness—can help you strengthen this alternative to autopilot and stay well. With practice, it's possible to change the habit of automatic "doing," realizing that "being" is always available in simple, routine moments of daily life.

What does autopilot or "doing mode" actually look or feel like in the context of everyday activities? Let's consider the example of Jan, who decided to practice mindfulness—moving from "doing" the daily activity of taking her prenatal vitamins to "being" present with her experience fully.

On autopilot or "doing mode," Jan described her experience like this: "I take my vitamins in the morning with breakfast. Sometimes I don't even notice that I've taken them, I'm so busy trying to get out the door, but a lot of times, as soon as I open the bottle, I'm thinking about whether I'm doing enough to be healthy during this pregnancy. I mean, I try to eat right and exercise, but I know I could be doing more. What if I'm not doing enough and it's hard on the baby? I think, 'I forgot to take my vitamin yesterday. What if the baby has some kind of health problems that I could have prevented? Is taking vitamins really enough?' I end up swirling around in those worries."

When practicing mindfulness and "being" in the activity of taking her vitamins, Jan described the experience like this: "I noticed the colors of the bottle, the bright pinks and orange. I was aware of picking up the bottle and the sound of the vitamins as I turned the bottle on its side to open the cap. I noticed the scent of the vitamins as I inhaled at the opening of the bottle. I felt the firm smoothness of the vitamin as I poured it into my palm. As I brought the vitamin up to my mouth, I was aware of the thought, 'Will taking vitamins really help my baby be healthy?' and I noticed that I was focused on thinking instead of how the vitamin felt on my tongue. I noticed that I wanted to swallow and the coolness of the water that I drank."

In both cases, Jan did the same thing: taking her prenatal vitamins. When on autopilot, "doing" the task of taking her vitamins, Jan's attention was focused on doubting herself as a mother and worrying about her baby. Practicing mindfulness offered an alternative to ruminating about the past and worrying about the future.

Although not "easy," simply "being" and noticing what you see, feel, hear, smell, and taste during any activity constitutes mindfulness and can help you shift out of autopilot. As it did for Jan, "being mode" provides an anchor for your attention in your immediate, physical experience. We're not suggesting mindfully taking vitamins will guarantee immediate and concrete benefits like feeling peaceful or at ease. What we are saying, however, is that committing to this practice today, and in similar ways every day, makes it more likely that mindfulness will be available to you during challenges in the future when it really can help you stay well.

Over time, we'll help you bring the skill of mindfulness to difficult thoughts, emotions, and situations. Because these experiences so easily trigger automatic pilot (You know the times when your "buttons" get pushed!), even if you don't realize it until later, it can be helpful to strengthen your mindfulness skills in the context of less challenging, everyday activities— the mindful eating, drinking, and washing dishes of Lesson 1, taking vitamins like Jan, or changing the baby, among other routine activities. Committing to practice in the context of such activities helps to make mindfulness more available when you are faced with the kinds of challenges that may have caused stress or put you at risk for depression in the past. Mindfulness can be a powerful ally in navigating conflicts with family or at work, dealing with sleepless nights, responding to worries about the baby, and other challenging times. It takes practice to have that ally at the ready. As Jon Kabat-Zinn, American professor emeritus of medicine and creator of the mindfulness-based stress reduction program, has said, "Weave your parachute every day; don't wait until you need to jump out of the plane."

Daily Practice for Lesson 2

To build your awareness of autopilot, we invite you to practice, at least once a day, catching yourself when you're on autopilot. Have you gotten to one place or activity from another without noticing the transition? Have you had your "buttons pushed" or reacted with strong emotion without realizing how you got so upset? Have you missed out on simple moments like seeing a friend smile or hearing your baby laugh or been aware of them only vaguely because your attention was elsewhere?

◆ Identify any situation in which you are on autopilot and record what you noticed in your Practice Journal at the end of this chapter.

◆ Briana describes times that she was on autopilot while doing this daily practice: "I literally drive the same road every day between work and dropping my kids off at day care. This week, I started paying attention to times that I was on autopilot, and I noticed that is true for most of my morning routine. So I started to catch myself as I was saying good-bye to the kids at day care. I noticed more as I was driving to work and realized there was a park with a playground back from the street just two blocks before my work. I never even saw that before; I was so much on autopilot.

It really struck me how much it's possible to miss if I didn't even see that park after driving that road every day for months!"

♦ Like Briana, you might notice things in your physical environment when you catch yourself on autopilot, or new emotions, thoughts, sensations, or experiences of other people around you. We're curious about what you will notice when you start catching autopilot!

Lesson 3. At Home in the Body

How easy is it for you to check in with your body and really know how you're feeling? If you asked yourself right now whether you are feeling fatigued or relaxed, had any aches or pains, how easy or challenging would you find it to answer accurately? Take a minute to try this:

Practice Now

Sitting (or lying down if you're reading in that position) comfortably, take a few slow, deep breaths, and feel yourself release tension with each exhale. Now bring your attention to the top of your head and simply feel whatever sensations are there. Tingling? Itching? Pulsing? Or maybe you notice an absence of sensation?

Very slowly, let your attention move down the front of your face. Be aware of whatever you encounter—tightness, relaxation, pressure. Is the sensation in your forehead, nose, mouth, and cheeks pleasant, painful, or neutral? Is your jaw clenched, loose, or knotted?

What did you discover? Maybe you were surprised to realize you had a slight headache. Or you were pressing your lips tightly together. Or your eyelids felt heavy. Or perhaps you experienced how challenging it can be to direct your attention without its wandering off.

You've just had a taste of a mindfulness practice called the body scan. Now imagine what it would be like to be able to shift your awareness fully to your belly if you felt a twinge that alarmed you or that little pleasant bubbling, fluttering sensation that many women describe when their baby starts to move in the second trimester of pregnancy.

Awareness of the body can help us focus on where we are right now, without trying to resist the feelings or prolong them, without the overlay of thoughts that keep us from the full experience of what the body is telling us. This awareness can tell you whether something is wrong that needs to be addressed to protect your health or that of your baby, but it can also tell you whether you're slipping into depression, dealing with too much stress or anxiety.

So many of us have trained ourselves to ignore the hunger pangs that tell us to pause and have lunch or the fatigue that tells us to pause and take a break. Often we rely on this capacity to stifle awareness of how our bodies are feeling. It can help us get things done. Now we might feel hyperaware at times—like when we're suddenly stopped in our tracks by a Braxton Hicks contraction, a round ligament pain, or, postnatally, the letdown reflex that takes us by surprise when someone *else's* baby cries within earshot. We also might feel clueless at other times, because we can't wrap our head around the idea that carrying around a growing, moving fetus makes us feel different from before.

With all these new sensations coming at you, now is a great time to reacquaint yourself with your body. It's uniquely equipped to keep you in touch with where you are right now—in this place, at this time, in this mental, emotional, and physical state. Listening to your body, as you will practice doing throughout this program, can help you take charge of your own well-being.

Our eight classes will give you an opportunity to practice with many formal mindfulness practices, which work hand-in-hand with the informal practices like mindfully eating and playing with your baby. Today we begin with our first formal practice, the body scan.

The Body Scan. We invite you to practice the full body scan. To prepare, it's important to choose a place to practice where you feel protected, comfortable, and warm. You can do this practice sitting in a chair or lying down in your bed or on a mat on the floor in a way that will be comfortable. If you're lying down, you can lay your arms alongside you, palms open to the ceiling if that feels comfortable to you. If you're pregnant, you may want to lie on your side, with pillows supporting your back and belly. What matters most is finding a position in which you are relaxed and supported, and this is likely to change from day to day throughout your pregnancy and early parenting. Because the body scan is a practice of being awake rather than falling asleep, it might be helpful to practice with your eyes open from time to time, especially if you are lying down and feelings of drowsiness arise.

We will scan the entire body with our attention, from top to bottom, exploring sensations and paying attention to whatever is happening, moment by moment, in the body.

Your attention may wander as you do this practice. We want to assure you that it's the nature of the mind to wander and to think. It is bound to happen a lot. This is not a sign that you are doing anything wrong. It's simply the mind on autopilot, thinking, judging, remembering, planning, and so forth. At these times, gently bring your attention back to the instructions and follow along as best you can.

If you have a baby growing within and you feel movements of the baby at any time during the practice, allow your attention to move to those sensations. During these times, you may allow your focus on the instructions to fade into the background and stay with the sensations of the baby moving. In this way, we encourage you to allow the baby to be your teacher, guiding you back to the present moment. As you will discover increasingly over time, your baby can be a powerful mindfulness teacher through pregnancy, labor, delivery, and all through your years of parenting. When you feel movement, bring your attention there, and when the movements subside, return to the instructions.

Practice Now

Once you have prepared your space, listen to "The Body Scan" (Track 5) to do this practice now. When you are finished, please return to reflect on your experience.

Reflections on Practice

What sensations did you notice while doing the body scan?

_____

_____

_____

_____

_____

Circle of Mothers

"I didn't notice many sensations because I just fell asleep. Or maybe I just zoned out. During the parts when there weren't guiding instructions and it was quiet, I was like half asleep . . . and then the voice would kind of come back and I'm thinking, I can't remember where we are in the body."

"I noticed the toes on my right foot feel really tingly."

"I think I spent the entire time thinking about an argument that my mother and I had last night. I felt some sensations in my face, but then I was pretty focused on this thing with my mom. I felt impatient and I wanted the instructions to end so that I could call my sister. I kept having to bring my attention back to the instructions again and again."

How did the experience of paying attention to your body in this practice differ from your typical experience of your body?

_____

_____

_____

_____

Circle of Mothers

"I kept thinking that I was doing it wrong. I was really distracted and impatient. I kept wondering if I should be doing it differently than I was."

"I have a lot of pressures in my life right now, so for me it was a very pleasant kind of quieting experience. It made me realize how busy I must have been all day, or maybe just in general. To sit still and kind of let other things go, I realize there are just a lot of things racing through my head on a normal day-to-day basis, so to not pay attention to it was really kind of nice. It felt peaceful . . . there was no TV, nobody talking. And I could feel the baby move a lot, kicking and flipping around."

"I don't think I really feel my body all that often. I think about my body a lot, like how much weight I'm gaining each week of this pregnancy, and whether it's too much or too little, but I don't really feel it all that much. This was different. I noticed tightness in my shoulders and a general feeling of drowsiness in my body."

As you reflect on your vision for staying well during pregnancy, postpartum, and beyond, described on page 19, how might this practice support you along the staying-well path?

_____

_____

_____

_____

Circle of Mothers

"I think that paying more attention to my body can help me become aware of stress and anxiety before it becomes a dark hole I disappear into. I think that this practice also can help me feel more in touch and present with the baby growing inside of me, which is something I've been having difficulty with thus far. It has felt so abstract and strange, and I've felt bad that I'm not more connected to the whole experience of being pregnant. I want to be connected to the feelings of being pregnant and to be close with my baby when she is born."

"I have been so busy since starting back to work. I was really stressing about going back to work, and it has been hard. My husband has been on me about doing some practices. I find that the body scan has been most helpful. I need him to kind of push me to do it at night, but when he does, I go into our bedroom and shut the door and listen to it on my phone while he watches the baby. I am shocked at how easy it is to let go of the stress of all that I am doing. I just lie there on the bed and listen to the instructions and feel my feet or my heart beating or whatever it is. I like that it's so concrete and clear. I just follow it along, and it really helps when I do it. I focus on what I'm actually feeling in my body instead of all these thoughts and pressures about what I have to get done and how I'm going to take care of everyone and everything."

Be Curious. In noticing sensations, thoughts, or emotions, it's helpful to be curious. Inquire of your experience: At what point did sensations arise? What was their quality, and in what ways did they shift over time? To what extent did intensity of the thoughts and images shift over time? No matter what the experience—pleasant, unpleasant, intense, or subtle—you can bring questions of interest and curiosity.

It's Okay to Feel Whatever You Feel. You might feel calm and relaxed during the body scan practice or a sense of restlessness, agitation, or boredom. Remember that whatever you experience is okay. The aim is simply to focus your attention on each part of the body in turn and notice the sensations that greet you. It is important to give yourself permission to let yourself feel what is arising in your body—whatever it is. The pregnant and postpartum body can be hard to live in. If you detect a sensation that's pleasant, you may feel a tendency to hang on to it. If so, you can practice letting go, opening, and seeing if you can be with the sensation of pleasure without trying to sustain it. If you detect a sensation that's unpleasant or uncomfortable, you may reflexively try to push it away; you may feel angry about it or afraid of it. If you spot any of these reactions, remember that you can notice them and let them go. The option always exists to come back to the direct experience of the moment—get curious about what is the actual sensation. Feel it directly, welcome it, as best you can. Practice being at home in your body, whatever you feel.

Don't Be Surprised by Self-Critical Thoughts. The majority of women struggle with critical thoughts about their bodies. Being pregnant and in the postpartum period can make these types of thoughts louder and more frequent. The invitation to focus on your body in this practice might be the last thing you want to do. This might be even more true for women who have struggled with weight or problems like binge eating, bulimia, or anorexia. The practice is inviting you to take a very different approach to your body, one that is gentle and friendly, emphasizing noticing sensations as they arise. Self-critical thoughts about your body might arise so intensely that they take center stage. Over the next few lessons, we will be learning a range of practices to help with such powerful thoughts. For now, know that many women find that bringing attention to the body opens the door to a flood of self-critical thoughts. As best you can, bring your attention back to the guiding instructions and the sensations you feel.

Let Your Experience Be Your Most Important Guide. Remember that you are in charge of how you practice. If it's helpful for you to break the practice into smaller units that you do in multiple sessions throughout the day, that is totally fine (e.g., your head and shoulders in the morning, your torso in the afternoon, and your lower body in the evening). What matters is beginning to shift your relationship with your body so that it can become a source of information and wisdom for you over time. If you have had many years (decades, even!) of a judgmental and critical relationship with your body, small steps of connecting differently with your body might make the most sense. There is no right or wrong way to do the body scan practice or this entire program.

It's Never Too Late to Begin Again. Each time you notice your attention pulled away by thoughts, whatever they might be, you have another opportunity to practice noticing and then to begin again. We invite you to bring your attention back to the guiding instructions, even if you have been pulled into thinking (or dozing off) for some time. Remember: it's never too late to begin again.

Your Body Is an Anchor to the Present Moment. The body can help to anchor our awareness in the present moment, not the past or future, and offers a way of stepping out of the autopilot of thinking, judging, and evaluating. This practice trains your ability to stay connected with how you are feeling in your body, moment to moment. It also trains your ability to direct your attention, rather than having autopilot carry you along without your awareness (or your consent!). As you move your attention to different parts of your body, you gain practice directing your attention on purpose.

Daily Practice for Lesson 3

Do the body scan once each day this week.

♦ Use "The Body Scan" (Track 5) to guide your practice. Once you have practiced the body scan with the audio instruction many times, you may choose to practice without the audio. Many women find that Sharon's voice sets the right tone for letting whatever arises emerge freely, and so they continue to use it.

◆ Give yourself permission to feel whatever you find as you move your attention throughout the body, following the instructions. As best you can, let go of the habits to hold on to pleasant sensations and push away unpleasant sensations. Allow your experience to be as it is, at home in your body, whatever you find. Even if you find yourself judging yourself or the practice, keep following the instructions.

◆ Briefly record the sensations, thoughts, or emotions that you notice in your Practice Journal at the end of the chapter after each practice.

Daily Practice Summary

To recap, we invite you to do the following daily practices and record your experiences in your Practice Journal below.

Lesson 1

• Practice mindful eating, drinking, or washing dishes at least once each day. You may use Tracks 1–4 for guidance the first few days and then continue on your own or with the ongoing support of the audio guidance. In short and simple responses, record what you notice in your Practice Journal.

Lesson 2

• To become aware of autopilot, at least once a day, practice catching yourself when you're on autopilot. Identify these situations and record what you notice in your Practice Journal.

Lesson 3

• Do the body scan each day, using "The Body Scan" (Track 5) for guidance. Record in the Practice Journal each time you listen to the guided body scan instructions, recording briefly the sensations, thoughts, or emotions that you notice.

Circle of Support

On at least one day, talk with your support person about what you learned from this chapter and what you are noticing in your daily practices. Record any reflections based on these conversations in the Circle of Support Reflections.

Practice Journal

	Day 1	Day 2	Day 3
Lesson 1 Practice: What did you notice during your mindfulness of everyday activities practice (eating, drinking tea, washing dishes)?			
Example: *I focused on eating a half peanut butter and raspberry jam sandwich for lunch. I loved noticing the sensation of the creamy peanut butter texture interspersed with the seeds in the raspberry jam. It was like there were these little surprises in the sandwich.*			
Lesson 2 Practice: Where/when did you catch yourself on autopilot today?			
Example: *I realized that I was on autopilot in the shower before going to bed. I was thinking about a ton of other things: making lists, thinking about work, etc. I was going through the motions of showering when I noticed that I wasn't really present for any of it. When I brought myself to the present in that space, I realized how wonderful it felt to stand under the warm water and relax, taking in deep breaths with the steam of the shower around me.*			
Lesson 3 Practice: What did you notice in your body scan practice today? What thoughts, sensations, or emotions were present?			
Example: *The feeling of frustration kept coming up for me and pulling me away from the guiding instructions. I kept wanting the practice to be quicker than it was. I was also so judgmental of my body. I kept coming back to the instructions, and it helped me notice that I was so tense in my shoulders, back, and legs. I kept reminding myself to release the tension and not wind myself up so tightly.*			

Practice Journal

Day 4	Day 5	Day 6	Day 7

Circle of Support Reflections

What did you notice in connecting with your support person this week?

CLASS 2

Body, Mind, and Breath

To pay attention, this is our endless and proper work.
—Mary Oliver

This chapter focuses on the following key lessons:

1. **Various challenges may arise during the body scan practice, but there are ways to greet these obstacles as opportunities for new learning.** We help you learn to work skillfully with challenges.

2. **The mind has a tremendous capacity to make interpretations, and it's helpful to understand the ways in which thoughts and feelings are connected.** We help you identify these connections. Because identifying our thoughts and feelings takes practice, we also expand our mindfulness of daily activities to include pleasant experiences and new activities, focusing, in particular, on labeling sensations, thoughts, and emotions.

3. **An important friend in learning to practice mindfulness is the breath.** We invite you to begin mindfulness of breathing with a brief daily practice.

Lesson 1. We Begin with the Body

There is more to our experience than the stories the mind is telling us. If you are vulnerable to feeling down or overwhelmed, the stories your mind tells often follow a common theme: negative and unchanging.

Often, the mind ignores neutral or positive information. Not only does the mind lock into what's negative in the here-and-now, but it also suggests things will always be that way. These stories your mind tells can send you down a slippery slope to feeling depressed or anxious.

The good news is that you can learn skills that help you stop the descent on the slippery slope. You don't have to slide down into feeling depressed or overwhelmed, even if that's where your mind's stories usually send you.

At these times, you have another option. You can anchor in the body instead of getting stuck in your head. Anchoring in your body gives you a way to keep autopilot on "off."

This is why practicing the body scan repeatedly—as you have been doing for the last week and will do again today—is such an important vehicle for learning mindfulness and staying well.

Anchoring in the body is useful for people vulnerable to depression or anxiety, and it is particularly valuable during pregnancy and postpartum. Pregnant and postpartum bodies are powerful teachers that things are in fact always changing. We undergo changes both visible (e.g., the size of the belly) and invisible (e.g., hormone levels). Connecting with these experiences can provide a counterpoint for some of the stories of the mind.

Consistent practice of the body scan helps in these ways:

- Opens your awareness to aspects of your experience beyond the stories your mind tells.

- Keeps autopilot from taking over.

- Allows you to practice moving attention in a deliberate way (repeatedly engaging, holding, and releasing).

- Teaches you about the changing nature of experience.

Practicing the body scan over the last 7 days may already have revealed to you some of these benefits.

Practice Now

We invite you to approach this body scan practice with a sense of newness and curiosity about what you will discover today. Take a few moments to prepare your space, and when you are ready, do the body scan, along with the recorded instructions on "The Body Scan" (Track 5) if you prefer. When you are finished, please return to reflect on your experience.

Reflections on Practice

What sensations did you notice while doing the body scan?

_____

_____

_____

_____

_____

"I was really focused in the first part, and I noticed the sensations of my pants against my ankles and then the muscles in my leg. Then the sound of a dog barking outside. It was so noisy, and it kept going and going. It was hard to concentrate!"

"My heartburn was so bad. It was really hard to pay attention to anything else, and it was hard to focus on that area too because mostly I just wanted to do something to make the discomfort from the reflux go away."

How did the experience of paying attention to your body in this practice differ from your typical experience of your body?

_____

_____

_____

_____

_____

"I know this is a time to take care of me and will help me manage my stress and anxiety, but my mind was racing so much of the time with my to-do list. I have a million things I need to do before this baby comes. I realize that this is how I am a lot of the time these days, always racing around and not really paying attention to what I'm feeling."

"I noticed the baby moving around during part of the practice. It was really sweet. Often I might notice when she moves but I don't really have time to focus on it. It was really nice to just pay attention to it."

"I gave myself a hard time during the whole practice. I just kept thinking 'I'm so selfish,' asking my mom to watch the baby so I can lie here doing nothing. That's kind of a usual story for me; my mind gives me a hard time a lot."

As you reflect on your vision for staying well during pregnancy, postpartum, and beyond, described on page 19, how might this practice support you along the staying-well path?

_____

_____

_____

_____

_____

_____

Circle of Mothers

"I fell asleep after about 1 minute. I've been up with the baby so much lately. I'm just exhausted. I think I slept through the whole thing. This is really connected to staying well for me because paying attention to whether I'm tired or hungry or whatever often is hard for me. Often I am not even aware of how tired I am. But these are the kinds of things that make a big difference in staying well."

"I was feeling okay when I started, but then it was like waves of anxiety came crashing down. I started to get really pulled into worrying about the amnio test next week. Then I listened to your instructions about letting go of thoughts and worries and refocusing on my body. I focused on the feeling of the temperature of the air in the room on my face, and I did notice that the worries got a little quieter. Not like they were gone, but more like they were in the background. I can see how this would help me over time."

Greeting Challenges as Opportunities

The body can be a great anchor and teacher when you are pregnant or postpartum because so much is happening and changing. At the same time, anchoring in the body can be particularly challenging during these times in a woman's life. The body faces major demands such as labor and delivery, sleeplessness, and other physical experiences.

Like the mothers in the circle, you likely experienced some challenges with the body scan. We invite you to consider how you can greet challenges as opportunities for strengthening your skills of mindfulness.

Review the table below to check off the challenges that were present for you in your experience just now or over the 7 days of your body scan practice. Once you have completed the checklist, please go back to each of the challenges that you experienced and consider the guidance for how to greet each one as an opportunity.

Check if true for you	Challenges	Greeting challenges as opportunities
____	Discomfort in the body	When we experience discomfort in the body, many of us find ourselves dwelling on the experience or working hard to make it go away. Doing so can carry you far from the moment-to-moment experience in the body. This pattern can be particularly troublesome given the myriad uncomfortable sensations that come with pregnancy, labor and delivery, and the postpartum. The body scan invites you to notice when your mind begins to wander in this way in response to uncomfortable sensations and to bring awareness back, as best you can, to the part of the body currently under focus in the instructions. This allows you to practice untangling yourself from the mental webs that autopilot can weave in response to discomfort. When the instructions guide your focus to the area of discomfort, explore the sensations with gentleness. Then, when guided to move to a new area, release the area of discomfort and move on.
____	Sleepiness	Pregnant, postpartum, and early parenting moms are often exhausted. Lying down in a comfortable, quiet, and warm place invites much needed sleep. If you experience this, know you are not alone. There is no need to add self-judgment to an exhausted body! Noticing how tired you are may be a helpful step itself in learning to care for yourself and stay well. At the same time, because the body scan is actually a practice of being awake to your experience, you might explore practicing with your eyes open from time to time if you are lying down and feelings of drowsiness arise. You might also explore whether other times of day or places to practice help you stay alert.

Check if true for you	Challenges	Greeting challenges as opportunities
____	Environmental conditions	Pregnancy, labor and delivery, and parenting teach us that it is impossible to control or even anticipate all environmental conditions. At times, things will not be the way you want them to be, and there is nothing you can do to change that. For example, the doctor or midwife with whom you are most connected is not on call when it is time to deliver your baby, or your baby is fussy and difficult to soothe when you have so much to do. Practicing the body scan can teach us how to remain connected to the present moment, even when it's not the moment we expected or prefer. For example, during the body scan, if you hear noises in the environment that are unpleasant (air conditioners, traffic, loud barking, children playing, TVs, etc.), you have an opportunity to name the experience (e.g., "hearing the TV") and your response (e.g., "annoyance is here") and return your attention to the instructions. This builds a skill that will come in handy when working with other challenging situations that arise during pregnancy or parenting.
____	Boredom	You might invite yourself to note the boredom as a state of mind in this moment and be curious about how you are responding to it. Did you notice yourself pushing away the experience of boredom as unwelcome? Did you notice yourself amplifying it by focusing on the aspects of the practice that bored you? Learning to tolerate and not get caught by boredom is important during pregnancy and early parenting. There are many moments of intensity in caring for a new baby, with emotional highs and lows. And there are many moments of boredom too. Practicing with the body scan now can help equip you with skills for these moments. As you practice, you might explore naming the boredom, perhaps gently noting to yourself "boredom is present," and then return to the instructions, bringing awareness back to the part of the body that is the intended focus, with curiosity for whatever you find.
____	Self-doubt or self-criticism	There is no right or wrong experience to have while doing the body scan practice. The intention is to bring gentle attention and curiosity to your experience, whatever it is, and to practice deliberately holding and shifting attention to different regions of the body. If you experience self-doubt, you might ask yourself: Am I comparing myself to some standard or expectation of how I think you "should" be feeling? And if I fall short of this expectation, am I responding with self-doubt or self-criticism? If so, you might explore reminding yourself that there is no one right way to feel, noticing that your attention was pulled away by thoughts of comparison, self-doubt, and self-criticism, and picking up with where the instructions guide. Also, you even might explore congratulating yourself for doing the

Check if true for you	Challenges	Greeting challenges as opportunities
		practice, no matter how it goes. This is great practice for being a mom, when we often have doubts and expectations about doing it "right"!
____	Mind wandering	If you notice that your mind has carried you far from the body, it's okay. It is not a sign that you are doing anything wrong. It's simply the mind on autopilot. You can easily pick up with where the instructions guide you. It's never too late to begin again. Nothing is lost. In fact, each time you practice responding gently and with kindness, returning your attention to the instructions, the skills of mindfulness are strengthened.
____	Relaxation	Experiencing the state of a peaceful and relaxed body can be delightful. It can be a gift to savor this experience when it occurs. This is especially true in this time of life when your body is working so hard, growing, birthing, caring for another human being! Creating time and space for relaxation and rest is critical. The body scan can provide a wonderful context to experience this. At the same time, remember that there is great value in the body scan, even when you do not feel relaxation at all. In fact, the body scan helps to strengthen the skill of paying attention to whatever is going on in the body—whether it is relaxation and ease or tension and tightness. This is a source of very important information, especially during this time of life when the body changes from day to day and moment to moment. For these reasons, we invite you to let go of expectations as you start the body scan each time, including the expectation that the practice will be relaxing. Enjoy the relaxation when it is present, and when it is not, know that it is valuable to practice being at home in the body and noticing what is there, whatever it is.
____	Difficult emotions	The body scan practice provides an opportunity to respond to difficult emotions, like sadness, anxiety, agitation, or frustration, in ways that may be different from how you usually respond to such emotions. In the context of the body scan, there is no need to do anything about these emotions, no need to fix or change them in any way. Instead, you are invited to allow them to arise, to acknowledge them, perhaps naming them as "sadness is here" if you find yourself crying during the practice, and to return awareness to the instructions. Doing so also allows you to continue to strengthen the skill of intentionally moving your attention, rather than being pulled completely into difficult emotions or the thoughts that go along with them. Over time, we will begin to work more directly with the negative emotions themselves, but at this point we encourage you to return to the instructions and focus on the body as a way of steadying yourself in the face of strong and difficult emotions that are so common during pregnancy and early parenting.

Check if true for you	Challenges	Greeting challenges as opportunities
_____	Doubt about the practice	It is normal and common for people at this point in the classes to have questions about the practices and the extent to which they will be helpful in cultivating well-being. You may be wondering, how will focusing on my knee help me stay well over time; how will it help me be the mom I want to be? Rather than tell you what will be helpful for you or what you should be doing, at this point in the program we encourage you to maintain an open mind and allow your own experience over time to respond to your doubts. We invite you to experience the body scan and the other practices enough to form your own opinions about how helpful each practice might be for you now and in the future. This capacity to keep an open mind and to learn from your own experience is particularly important for pregnant, postpartum, and parenting moms who get so much advice. Without the skill of attending to your own experience as an anchor, you can find yourself drowning in all of the opinions about how to be a "good" mother.
_____	Frustration about lack of time to do the practice	If you are wondering how it will be possible to add these practices to your busy life, you are not alone. We encourage you to prioritize time for practice during the weeks you have dedicated to this class. We also recognize that some days will be more challenging than others. The important thing is making the space and time to do the practice, even in a shortened way. So, if it comes to not having enough time to do the whole practice, we encourage you to do a shortened version of the practice. Shortening the practice or breaking up a practice over more than one practice period isn't wrong and it doesn't mean you are failing. It is not "against the rules." Watch out for the vicious cycle that can begin if you miss a practice time or day (or days) and begin to think you are "failing" at the course. Practicing being kind with yourself is as important a practice as any other practice you will learn in this class. Remember your motivation for learning these skills and come back, gently, to a brief practice as a way to begin again.

Being Curious and Gentle

How do you practice greeting challenges as opportunities? Let's consider the example of Marta, who struggled with drowsiness during the body scan practice.

When approaching her drowsiness as an obstacle, Marta said: "I'm not sure if I should keep doing this program. It's only the first week, and I've fallen asleep during every single one of the body scan practices. I don't know if it's the woman's voice being so soothing or if I'm just plain exhausted from being up with the baby, but I can't seem to stay awake past the part where you focus on the top of your head. I know the baby is up a lot, but other mothers seem to take it more in stride than I do. I see other moms at the play group, and they don't seem so wiped out."

After reading the experiences of other moms in the circle of mothers and the guidance about how to approach challenges as opportunities (starting on page 42 of this book), Marta shifted her approach to the drowsiness. She explained: "When I do the practice with the idea that all moms experience exhaustion at some point, it really shifts the experience. I am not so hard on myself. I give myself permission to feel the drowsiness without getting so freaked out if I happen to fall asleep. I remind myself that each time I practice is a new opportunity. I'm also more aware of how it feels to be tired, and I've started doing the practice in the living room instead of in my bed at times that I'm really wiped out. That helps me stay alert for a longer time in the practice. I still don't make it much past the belly, but I don't give myself a hard time about it as much. I think I'm going to keep going with this program and do it in whatever ways make sense in the moment; whether I fall asleep or stay awake isn't the most important thing."

With practice, Marta began to approach the same experience—exhaustion—as an opportunity. She interpreted her falling asleep as a common and understandable part of taking care of an infant. She also stayed connected to the sensations in her body in ways that allowed her to respond to what she needed, whether it was practicing in a new location that helped her stay awake longer or allowing herself to sleep as her body needed. When she responded to the exhaustion in these ways, she felt hopeful and empowered.

Review the rows of "challenges" you identified in the table above, select one, and reflect on ways in which you might begin to practice greeting it as an opportunity:

_____

_____

_____

_____

_____

Daily Practice for Lesson 1

Do the body scan once each day.

◆ It takes repeated practice to build new habits. For this reason, we continue with the body scan practice for each of the next 7 days. Continuing the body scan also helps you notice the changing nature of experience; we invite you to approach each practice session with openness and curiosity. Consider opportunities to greet challenges as teachers in the ways that we described in the table.

- ◆ You may use "The Body Scan" (Track 5) to guide your practice or practice without the audio.
- ◆ On each of the 7 days that you do the body scan, briefly record in your Practice Journal, at the end of this chapter, the sensations, thoughts, or emotions that you noticed and the ways in which you greet a challenge as an opportunity for learning.

Lesson 2. The Power of Interpretations

Marta's experience highlights the power of our interpretations about how we feel and what we do. We invite you to do a brief practice to understand this directly.

Practice Now

Settle into a comfortable position. Read through the paragraph below. In fact, you may want to read it over a couple of times to become fully familiar with the scenario.

You are walking down the street. On the other side of the street, you see someone you know. You have not seen this person since before you became pregnant. You smile and wave. The person just doesn't seem to notice and walks by.

When you are ready, we invite you to close your eyes and imagine yourself in that situation as vividly as possible. Then return to complete the following reflection questions.

- *What was the first thing that went through your mind as you imagined yourself in this situation?*

_____

_____

_____

- *What thoughts did you experience?* Thoughts are brief statements or images that come to mind.

_____

_____

- *What emotions did you experience?* Emotions can be described with one word: sad, mad, happy, afraid, ashamed, guilty, angry.

_____

_____

Circle of Mothers

Look at the following responses of the different mothers to exactly the same scenario. Notice the range of thoughts they experienced. Then draw a line between each thought and the emotion that might be shaped by that thought. Notice the ways in which the different thoughts connect to different emotions. There are no right or wrong answers here, and one emotion can fit more than one thought.

Thoughts	*Emotions*
Maybe something bad happened, and I don't know what it is.	Anxious
Did other people see me waving? How embarrassing!	
	Ashamed
I never told her I was pregnant; maybe she's upset with me because I didn't call her to tell her. I should have called her.	
	Guilty
She's probably mad at me; I'm going to lose all my old friends now that I'm having a baby.	
	Sad or down
I'm 8 months pregnant! How could she not have seen me? Forget her. I get so angry when people act like that. How rude!	
	Angry or frustrated
That was so nice to see her. What a pleasure to catch a glimpse of her after all these months, even though she didn't seem to see me. I want to give her a call when I get home.	
	Happy
She probably doesn't even recognize me; I'm such a mess now that all I do is take care of an infant 24 hours a day. I have gained so much weight, and I can barely remember when I last washed my hair!	

What surprises you in reviewing the range of thoughts and emotions?

_____

_____

_____

_____

Thoughts and Emotions

The thoughts above are each mother's individual interpretations of the situation, and such interpretations can have a powerful impact on how each mother feels. Often our emotions reflect our interpretations of a situation rather than the situation itself. The stories we tell ourselves can have a powerful effect on how we feel. A key lesson of this program is that thoughts are not facts—they are events in the mind. Also, these interpretations can often happen very quickly and, at times, even without awareness. So, one minute you may be walking down the street feeling fine, and the next minute you may have feelings of guilt come over you with little sense of how or why.

Filling in the Blanks

Automatically making interpretations often happens in ambiguous situations. Instead of allowing the ambiguity and seeking more information before drawing conclusions, the mind fills in the blanks—and if you are vulnerable to depression or anxiety, the mind fills in the blanks with negative interpretations and then responds to these interpretations as facts. During pregnancy and postpartum, you are likely to encounter many ambiguous situations. For example: Your doctor's office leaves you a message to call back without explaining why. Your results from a medical test are confusing or unclear. Your partner is staying late at work more than usual. Your baby may be giving you some signals you don't fully understand. If life in general provides plenty of ambiguous situations for us to interpret, pregnancy and parenting young ones provide more than one's fair share. If you are sleep-deprived, hungry, or stressed, as you often are during pregnancy, the postpartum, and early parenting, your mind may go to negative interpretations even more easily than at other times. Moreover, if you have experienced depression or anxiety in the past, you may be even more vulnerable to filling in the blanks with negative interpretations. Negative moods may make negative thoughts more likely, and negative thoughts may be early warning signs that depression or anxiety is returning.

Imagine now that you experienced the "walking down the street" scenario when you were feeling sleep-deprived, hungry, down, or anxious. Which of the thoughts or interpretations that you read from the circle of mothers (on the previous page) would be more likely to come to mind?

_____

_____

_____

_____

Everyday Experiences Provide Opportunities to Practice

It is not easy to become aware of our tendency to make rapid interpretations and to identify the connections between those interpretations and how we feel. Identifying our thoughts and feelings in response to different situations takes practice.

Starting with Pleasant Experiences

Paying attention to pleasant experiences can help you become aware of the specific components of your experience. Often people say, "It was a good day" or "I had a good time." Making interpretations like "good" or "bad" often happens without our awareness. In doing so, we often are not very connected to the components of such experiences. Paying attention to pleasant experiences can help you become more skilled at identifying the specific thoughts, emotions, and body sensations that make up what you categorize as "pleasant." This practice also helps you notice pleasant experiences that might otherwise escape your awareness. People with histories of depression can experience a pull of their attention to the negative, even when they are not depressed. The practice of noticing the pleasurable can help to bring a healthier balance to everyday life. As one mother reflected: "I often find myself rushing through my day with no real focus on what makes me happy. But ignoring the positive means that negative experiences typically take center stage. Focusing on pleasant experiences helped to improve my general mood all week. I was more balanced. I enjoyed thinking back on the pleasant moments at the end of the day, and I actually started to look forward to that part of the daily practice at the end of each day."

Daily Practice for Lesson 2

First Practice: At least once a day, for 7 days, pay attention to one pleasant experience, preferably while it's occurring.

- ◆ Remember that the pleasant experience can be simple and brief, such as feeling the sun on your face or seeing your baby sleeping peacefully.

- ◆ Use the Pleasant Experiences Practice Journal at the end of this chapter to record the components of your experience. Record thoughts as if you were saying them out loud, in the words that actually came into your mind, and describe emotions and body sensations in as much detail as possible.

Second Practice: Select one daily activity and make a deliberate effort to bring moment-to-moment awareness to that activity each time you do it.

◆ You can continue to use the audio instructions for the daily practices of "Drinking Tea Mindfulness," "Eating Mindfulness," or "Washing Dishes Mindfulness" (Tracks 2–4), or you can select another activity. There are many activities with which to practice during pregnancy and postpartum, so allow your own daily life to be your guide.

◆ Bring your awareness to what you are doing as you are actually doing it, noticing when you slip back into automatic pilot and then returning your attention to the daily activity as best you can. Record in your Practice Journal the activity you practiced mindfully each day.

◆ If you want to add a new activity and would like some suggestions, here is a list of some additional potential routine activities:

- First few breaths upon awakening
- Turning on a computer
- Drinking
- Listening to music
- Cooking
- Waking up in the morning
- Saying good morning/good night
- Getting into bed at night
- Using the phone
- Folding laundry
- Opening the car door
- Changing diapers
- Settling into a meeting at work
- Sweeping floors
- Scrubbing tubs
- Straightening up
- Taking out the garbage
- Driving
- Waiting in line
- Brushing teeth, bathing, showering
- Getting dressed
- Brushing/drying hair

Lesson 3. The Breath Is a Great Friend

What has been present since the moment of your birth, is with you all the time, and is something you can always rely on? Your breath. In learning to be mindful as a mother or mother-to-be, the breath can be a great friend.

In the coming classes, we will rely heavily on the breath as a focus for our formal meditation practice. This form of meditation doesn't require anything fancy or complex. It doesn't require you to sit in any certain postures or stop your thoughts. As long as you're breathing, you can learn this practice.

Mindful breathing provides us with skills that go everywhere with us and are available at all times. Whether it's at the supermarket or in the obstetrician's waiting room, while feeding a hungry baby or rocking a fussy one, the breath anchors us in the present moment.

The practice of mindful breathing has the potential to help us change the ways in which we respond to our own thoughts and emotions and to other people in our lives. Mindful breathing also can help us catch ourselves slipping into autopilot. When we first practice focusing attention on the breath, we quickly discover that our attention doesn't stay on the breath for very long! We may notice how often we are pulled away from the present moment. We may see habits of being, like talking to ourselves in harsh or critical ways, that don't serve us well during tough times. In these ways, the practice of mindful breathing can help us learn a great deal.

We're curious about what you will discover. In our next class, we will have an opportunity to explore in detail the practice of mindful breathing. Here we invite you to simply "meet" the breath in a 10-minute practice.

Practice Now

Choose a place that is comfortable for you and practice now with 10 minutes of mindful breathing. Listen to the "Introduction to Sitting" (Track 6) and then use the audio recording for the "10-Minute Breathing Meditation" (Track 7) to guide your practice. Once you've listened to the "Introduction to Sitting," you may choose to listen only to the "10-Minute Breathing Meditation" for future practices (Track 7).

Reflections on Practice

What did you notice while bringing your attention to the sensations of breathing?

_____

_____

_____

_____

Was the gentle noting of "breath, not breath" helpful to you? In what ways?

_____

_____

_____

_____

As you reflect on your vision for staying well during pregnancy, postpartum, and beyond, how might this practice support you along the staying-well path?

_____

_____

_____

_____

Daily Practice for Lesson 3

Practice mindfulness of breathing each day with the 10-minute breathing meditation.

♦ Listen to the "Introduction to Sitting" (Track 6).

♦ Use Track 7 to guide your daily mindful breathing practice. Once you've practiced with the audio instruction many times, you may choose to practice without the audio; however, most women find it to be helpful support in the beginning (and many continue to use it over time).

♦ Being with your breath for a few minutes each day provides an opportunity to become aware of what it feels like to be connected and present in the moment without having to do anything. It's an opportunity to step out of "automatic pilot" and "doing mode" and give yourself the gift of just being. In short and simple responses, record what you noticed in your Practice Journal.

Daily Practice Summary

To recap, we invite you to do the following daily practices and record your experiences in your Practice Journal.

Lesson 1

- Do the body scan each day and consider the opportunities to greet challenges as teachers in the ways that we described in the table (starting on page 43). Briefly record the sensations, thoughts, or emotions that you noticed and the ways in which you greeted a challenge as an opportunity for learning in your Practice Journal.

Lesson 2

- Notice and record the components of one pleasant event each day in your Pleasant Experiences Practice Journal.

- Select one daily activity and make a deliberate effort to bring moment-to-moment awareness to that activity each time you do it. Record the activity you experienced mindfully in your Practice Journal.

Lesson 3

- Practice 10 minutes of mindful breathing each day using Track 7 for guidance. Briefly record what you notice during your practice in your Practice Journal.

Circle of Support

- On at least one day, talk with your support person about what you learned from this chapter and what you're noticing in your daily practices. Record any reflections based on these conversations in your Circle of Support Reflections.

Practice Journal

	Day 1	Day 2	Day 3
Lesson 1 Practice Reflections: What did you notice in your body scan practice today? What thoughts, sensations, or emotions were present? In what ways did you greet a challenge as an opportunity for learning?			
Example: *I was a bit kinder to myself when my mind wandered or when I got bored, which still happened a lot. I told myself it's okay and then I would slowly come back to the instructions.*			
Lesson 2 Practice Reflections: Note each day the daily activity that you experienced mindfully. Record what activity you did each day.			
Example: *Eating dinner; it was one of the times I was most present in the day.*			
Lesson 3 Practice Reflections: What did you notice in your mindfulness of breathing practice?			
Example: *I did only the first few minutes of the recording because I had so much to do today. At first, mostly I felt irritated with the length of the recording. Then I noticed some sensations of tightness in my chest and belly.*			

Practice Journal

Day 4	Day 5	Day 6	Day 7

Pleasant Experiences Practice Journal

	Day 1	Day 2	Day 3
What was the experience?			
Example: *Sitting down on the couch at the end of a long day*			
What sensations in your body were present during the experience?			
Example: *Deep exhale while sinking into the couch, feeling the support of the cushions*			
What moods or feelings were present during the experience?			
Example: *Happy, content*			
What thoughts were present during the experience?			
Example: *It's such a relief to sit down.*			
What thoughts are in your mind now as you write this down?			
Example: *Small moments can make a big difference sometimes.*			

Pleasant Experiences Practice Journal

Day 4	Day 5	Day 6	Day 7

Circle of Support Reflections

What did you notice in connecting with your support person this week?

CLASS 3

Rhythms of Motherhood

Dance the rhythm of this moving world.
—Rumi

This chapter focuses on three key lessons, through which we introduce a number of practices for you to explore:

1. **You can be mindful in stillness and movement**. We invite you to discover this through sitting practices like mindfulness of breathing and movement practices like walking and yoga.

2. **The simple 3-minute breathing space practice is one that you can "carry in your pocket" and use throughout the day**. We invite you to integrate this practice as a routine part of your daily life.

3. **You can expand your practice of mindfulness to all sorts of situations that arise when pregnant or parenting, including the unpleasant ones**. We invite you to explore two new practices—the practice of "being with baby" and the practice of noticing unpleasant experiences—as ways to build on your practice of noticing routine daily activities and pleasant experiences.

We live in a fast-paced world. Pregnancy and motherhood don't change that, but they can definitely change the rhythm of our lives. You can feel like you're moving fast without a moment to pause for a breath and then find yourself sitting for hours holding a sleeping baby or caring for a sick child. Also, just when you develop a rhythm that you can handle, things change as the baby grows and develops, and schedules and routines shift rapidly from week to week, even day to day. If you're to make mindfulness a part of your daily, staying-well life, you'll need practices that are flexible and adaptable to a variety of circumstances, many of which can't be anticipated with any certainty.

To make mindfulness a dependable part of your routine, you also will need practices that can bring stillness in a busy or unpredictable day and practices that can help you work with a busy mind, even when you're sitting still and time seems to be dragging on. You need practices you can use at a moment's notice in the midst of whatever is going on around you, to help support you during pregnancy and early parenting.

Lesson 1. Mindful Stillness and Movement

There are many ways to practice strengthening the skill of mindfulness. The first part of today's class introduces three major practices: sitting meditation and two movement practices, walking and yoga.

Sitting Meditation

Teresa, pregnant with her second child, was starting to clean up the kitchen after settling her 2-year-old son into his high chair with a handful of cereal. It had been a challenging morning, and she was grateful for a chance to create a little more order by putting the dishes in the dishwasher. After a few minutes, her son started fussing, and she handed him his sippy cup with juice. Next thing she knew, he had flung the cup across the room, the lid flew off, and sticky apple juice splashed all over the cabinets and floor.

The experience and her response were all too familiar to her. She felt exhausted and angry. When she shared the story with us, though, she reported having felt surprised at what happened next: "I paused and took a breath. He was fussing, there was juice all over the floor, and I stood there, still, and breathed a few times. It wasn't long, and it might not seem like much, but it totally changed everything that followed." In the past, Teresa explained, she would have reacted automatically to her experience of frustration with a sharp tone with her son or throwing the cup, herself, into the sink. In this situation, her son would have escalated quickly from fussing to crying, and she would have been filled with thoughts about being a bad mother.

This time was different. Teresa had a tool to rely on—her breath. How did she develop the capacity to come to her breath in the midst of intense demands and emotions? The practice of sitting meditation is the training ground on which she developed the skills that allowed her breath to be a resource for her in the midst of the all-too-frequent challenges that pregnancy and parenting add to everyday life.

We had an opportunity to "meet" the breath in Class 2. Here we build on that with the practice of sitting meditation, which begins with a focus on the breath and expands to include a focus on sensations in the body and the experiences of hearing and thinking.

The essence of the sitting meditation practice is focusing on the feeling of the in-and-out breath and, later, expanding your awareness to include other objects of attention, such as sensations, hearing, and thinking.

Doing this practice doesn't require sitting in a certain posture or doing anything special or unusual. For the longer sitting practice that we invite you to do now, it helps if your back is straight, without being strained or overarched. Let yourself find a position that supports you in being alert but also allows you to have a sense of comfort and ease. You can practice on a chair or on the floor. If you use a chair, it can be helpful to use a straight-backed chair in which you can sit comfortably with your feet flat on the floor. If you choose to sit on the floor, you might find it helpful to sit on a firm cushion that allows you to sit 3–6 inches off the floor. Remember that what you need to feel a sense of support and ease may not be the same from day to day; the body changes throughout pregnancy and the postpartum, so take a few moments before beginning the practice to check in with how you are feeling and what positions or props will best support you today.

Practice Now

Choose a place that is comfortable for you and practice now with 25 minutes of mindful breathing. If you like, you may begin with reviewing the "Introduction to Sitting" (Track 6) and then use the audio recording for the "25-Minute Sitting Meditation" (Track 8) to guide your practice.

Reflections on Practice

What did you notice while doing the sitting practice?

_____

_____

_____

_____

Circle of Mothers

"I really felt the baby moving a lot. I loved that part of the practice. It was peaceful too, just focusing on my breathing."

"My back was killing me. It's been bothering me since the start of this trimester. I kept thinking about what I can do to feel better. It was hard to focus on much else."

What specific sensations did you notice (pressure or temperature in the body, pitch or volume in hearing, etc.)? In what ways did these sensations stay the same or change as you paid attention to them?

_____

_____

_____

_____

Circle of Mothers

"I noticed the rhythm of the air conditioning sound. It kind of came on and off. It reminded me of the mobile we're planning to get for the baby's room, so I started thinking about setting up the room for a while, but I came back to hearing the air conditioning sounds come and go."

What was the nature of the thoughts that arose? In what ways did your thoughts get drawn into the past or the future? Or to judging or blaming yourself? What was your experience of noticing thoughts like clouds moving through the sky?

_____

_____

_____

_____

Circle of Mothers

"I kept thinking about this argument with my mother-in-law, no matter how hard I tried not to think about it. Then I did the cloud thing. I imagined what I was thinking of saying to her and what she said to me like clouds and wind blowing them across the sky. That was really helpful. I felt more relaxed, and then I focused on my breathing after the thoughts passed."

As you reflect back on your vision for staying well during pregnancy, postpartum, and beyond, how might this practice support you along the staying-well path?

_____

_____

_____

_____

Circle of Mothers

"I know this is about taking care of my well-being, but I keep worrying this might not be enough and whether I can be a good mother when the baby comes. I do see that it's a really important part because I have really brief moments when I am focused on the present moment with my breathing. I can see how doing that more will help me be the kind of mom I want to be, even though it's a challenge."

The Breath as a Friend

Like these mothers, you may discover the ways in which the breath can help to anchor you in the present moment. You also may notice how active the mind can be when you bring stillness to the body. The mind is easily pulled into the past or the future, whereas the breath is always available as a focus of attention in the present moment. Focusing attention on breathing is a skillful alternative to having your attention pulled into the past or the future. For those who are vulnerable to depression, stress, or anxiety, often the mind gets stuck in negative thoughts or images from the past or worries about the future. Some of these thoughts can be very powerful, hijacking your attention and carrying you into depression. Practicing sitting meditation each day helps you become more familiar with the breath as a purposeful focus of attention. In this way, the breath can be a great friend that is available as an anchor, no matter where you are.

Regardless of what is happening in the mind, the breath can be a safe place to which you can return. Remember that the practice is one of noticing the sensations of breathing in the body—at the nostrils, chest, or belly. There is no need to control the breath, to make it deep, even, relaxed, or anything else. Simply allow your body to breathe and notice the moment-by-moment experience of breathing.

How to Respond When the Mind Is Very Busy

You may discover that your mind is very active and busy at some times, perhaps pulled to negative thoughts but also to positive or even neutral thoughts. It is the nature of the mind on autopilot to travel in these ways. During pregnancy or with a new baby, there are so many sensations in the body, emotions, and demands that pull for your attention.

When your mind wanders during your sitting meditation practice, the invitation is to begin again by gently redirecting your attention to the chosen focus. It's okay if you redirect your attention many times. In fact, it's important to remember that each sitting meditation practice invites you to do the following:

1. Select a point of focus for your attention (e.g., the breath).
2. Maintain your awareness on this point of focus.

3. Notice when your attention has wandered to another focus point (e.g., thinking about the mobile for the baby's room), let go of attending to the new point of focus (e.g., disengage attention from the image of the mobile), and gently return your attention to the original point of focus (e.g., the breath).

Many people think that the practice of mindfulness is only Step 2, but each of the steps above is essential. In fact, the place where people often struggle—Step 3—is a great opportunity to practice being gentle with yourself. You are not failing if your mind wanders. It takes practice to step out of autopilot.

Let's say you're focusing on the breath during sitting meditation, and suddenly your attention wanders to thoughts of a phone call you forgot to return. In fact, you don't just remember the phone call; your mind is halfway through envisioning the conversation with the other person when you notice, "Oh, my attention has wandered. It's not on the breath." The experience of letting go of the phone call in this moment is a powerful way to strengthen your skill of mindfulness. "So what?" you might ask, "Who cares about letting go of thoughts about a trivial phone call?"

Practicing letting go of these seemingly unimportant thoughts (or sensations) that arise during your meditation practice is the very same skill that can help you let go of ruminative, painful thoughts like "I'm not a good mother." It is the very same skill that helped Teresa respond differently to her son throwing the apple juice all over the floor. The practice of meditation allows us to build our skill with letting go of more neutral thoughts like "I forgot to return that phone call," so that we are ready to learn how to protect ourselves from getting hijacked by the more difficult ones. In Class 4, we focus more directly on these types of difficult thoughts; for now, we focus on building a strong foundation of mindfulness practice.

Mindful Movement

As we noted earlier, to make mindfulness a reliable part of life, most women find value in both the stillness in sitting meditation and the movement in practices like walking and yoga. In this part of Lesson 1, we introduce you to these practices and invite you to explore one right now and both during your daily practice this week.

Alyssa, pregnant with her second child, was clear in our first class that her main focus was learning skills to cope with stress and anxiety. When others spoke of noticing "busy minds" during the sitting practice, she often laughed that her mind was on "overdrive" with planning and worrying. She had struggled with the sitting practice, both with finding time to do it as a pregnant mom with a 4-year-old and a full-time job and with feeling distracted and agitated during the practice. She immediately embraced the idea of movement practices. Yoga and walking, she found, helped settle her mind and inspired her to weave these practices into her day.

In addition, she realized quickly what little awareness she had of her body while her attention was captured by her worrying mind. As she practiced noticing how she felt in her body while moving her arms above her head during one of the yoga postures, she became aware of the tension in her neck and shoulders. She commented after the practice: "I'm always talking about how my body is changing with this pregnancy, gaining weight and all that, but I really hadn't been paying attention to how my feelings in my body are connected to how I'm feeling emotionally. I'm certainly aware of being anxious a lot of the time, but I didn't realize how much my muscles are tense and tight and how exhausted I feel physically. When I'm overly focused on my worries, I put all my time into trying to fix them, but being more aware of my body helps me remember that I need to take care of myself right now and bring a little more comfort or rest to all this tension I feel physically."

Like Alyssa, many of us spend much more time focused on what's happening "in our heads," such as thoughts of a conflict with a family member or what's next on a long list of things "to do." We may miss the information that is available in the body about how we are feeling and what is important to our well-being.

Alyssa returned to our third class, excited to share two ways in which she was grateful for the movement practice. The first wasn't a surprise; she said: "The walking really helps with its focus on action and moving. It keeps my mind from thinking too much about details. If I allow myself a few minutes for walking, I notice it's easier for me to settle into a sitting practice and focus on my breathing." For many women, mindful movement can be particularly helpful when feeling agitated or anxious. Mindful movement can settle a busy mind, similar to soothing a fussy baby through gentle rocking movements.

The second was a pleasant surprise for her and us. Alyssa described doing the yoga practice at home one evening and realizing that it was possible to do the yoga with her 4-year-old daughter. She explained: "This week, I discovered that I could do the yoga with her, and she really loved it. I don't feel as much of a conflict with finding time for practice, and that, in and of itself, is a big relief. Plus, it's kind of given us a fun common ground that brings us closer. And it's super helpful to feel like I'm taking what I'm learning and passing it on to my daughter."

We're curious about what you will discover in your own practice of mindful yoga or walking, especially when you begin to notice the effects on your body and mind.

The Practice of Yoga

Yoga has become increasingly popular in recent years, particularly among pregnant and postpartum women. It is a practice that can be used in daily life. You don't need elaborate equipment or years of training to reap its benefits. Many people practice yoga simply as a form of physical exercise. A regular practice of yoga can lead to improvements in physical flexibility, balance, and strength, and recent research suggests that yoga practice also may have specific health benefits among pregnant women, including labor and delivery outcomes. Although these are important, they are not the only benefits of a yoga practice. In this class, we practice yoga as a form of mindful movement. Practicing in this way can help you become more aware of sensations in the body, thoughts, emotions, and the relationship among them and can help you ride the ever-changing rhythms in each day of pregnancy or early parenting.

As with any mindful movement, it is important to be patient with and listen to your own body. This practice is not about achieving or doing more, but about noticing and observing what's already here, without judging or criticizing yourself. Take care not to overstretch and to be gentle with yourself, even though your flexibility increases during pregnancy. If a pose does not feel right for you, don't do it. Listening to your body and your moment-to-moment experience is the most important instruction in this practice (and this entire course!). *Do not force yourself into any of the poses.*

Walking Meditation

Walking is a very common form of exercise among pregnant women. It's also something most mothers find themselves doing a lot with newborns. Walking meditation presents you with lots of opportunities to bring mindfulness into what is likely already an everyday activity for you. Unfortunately, many of us often walk on autopilot. We're walking to get from place to place, and often our attention is completely consumed by what we'll say or do when we get there or perhaps thoughts of something that just happened. We miss the actual experiences of walking, whatever those experiences might be. The essence of walking meditation is to bring mindfulness to this act that we normally do mechanically and without awareness.

In this exercise, you are invited to bring your attention into the body, to bring awareness to this activity of movement. We do this practice with our eyes open, and the awareness we bring to the body is a light awareness. You can be in touch with the sensations in your body even as you are aware of what's going on around you—what you're seeing and hearing. In the midst of the wider awareness of what's going on around you, you also have this touchstone, this center of awareness in your body.

Practice Now

Now we invite you to learn from you own experience of mindful movement. Select either the yoga or walking practice to explore right now (or you are welcome to explore both today!). You will have an opportunity to practice with each during this week's daily practices.

If you select the walking, listen to the "Walking Meditation" recording (Track 9).

If you select the yoga, please watch the 1-minute "Yoga Introduction" (Video 1) and then practice along with the "10-Minute Yoga Practice" (Video 2). These practices were recorded with pregnant women, so they are appropriate for prenatal use; however, they are equally important for women during early parenting.

When you're finished, please return to reflect on your experience.

Reflections on Practice

What did you notice while doing the mindful movement practices?

_____

_____

_____

Circle of Mothers

"At first, I was mostly aware of my thoughts. I kept thinking about this ultrasound I have scheduled for tomorrow. As I started the yoga, my thoughts started to slow down. I realized I was clenching my jaw and my shoulders were really tense. As I paid attention to my feet on the ground, my body relaxed a little more. I felt my shoulders drop down a bit after I lifted them up and down."

In what ways was your experience of mindful movement similar to or different from your experience of movement in everyday life?

_____

_____

_____

_____

Circle of Mothers

"Sometimes when I'm walking my baby at night, I'm just saying to him, in my mind, over and over, "Go to sleep; stop crying." When I did this practice with him, I noticed those thoughts were starting up like they usually do. Then I reminded myself to come back to focus on the walking. I repeated the word 'lifting' each time I took a step. The thoughts were still there, kind of in the background, but I wasn't as focused on them. I was still exhausted, but I wasn't as stressed out."

As you reflect on your vision for staying well during pregnancy, postpartum, and beyond, how might this practice support you along the staying-well path?

_____

_____

_____

Circle of Mothers

"The yoga was really hard for me. I kept thinking about how much weight I've gained and how hard it is to move around now. Those postures would have been not a big deal before this pregnancy. I just kept thinking, 'I'm so out of shape; how is it that I haven't lost more weight since the baby came?' I wanted to push myself, but I remembered the instruction about not forcing yourself. I realize that it's hard for me to be gentle with myself. Getting more practice with that would help with the yoga and with being less critical with myself as a new mom."

Daily Practice for Lesson 1

Do a practice each day, alternating between the sitting practice and the yoga or walking movement practices. You may select either the yoga or walking practice on the movement day, or you may do both on those days.

- Sitting meditation: Days 1, 3, 5, and 7. Practice with 25 minutes of mindful breathing. If you like, you may begin with reviewing the "Introduction to Sitting" (Track 6) and then use the audio recording for the "25-Minute Sitting Meditation" (Track 8) to guide your practice. On days in which it's challenging to make time for the 25-minute practice, the "10-Minute Breathing Meditation" may be a helpful option (Track 7).

- Yoga or walking practice: Days 2, 4, and 6. If you select the yoga practice, use the "25-Minute Yoga Practice" instructions (Video 3). On especially busy days, you might rely on the "10-minute Yoga Practice" (Video 2). If you select the walking practice, please listen and practice along with the 8-minute "Walking Meditation" instructions (Track 9). You can do the walking practice indoors or out, although it may be easier to practice indoors the first few times.

- Briefly record in your Practice Journal the sensations, thoughts, or emotions that you notice each time you practice.

Lesson 2. The 3-Minute Breathing Space

Have you ever sat in the waiting room before a prenatal or pediatrics appointment feeling anxious about what's to come? Have you ever found yourself up in the middle of the night, exhausted and feeling at your wit's end? Have you ever been sitting in traffic with a crying baby in the car seat? In the heat of such moments, does it seem that mindfulness is out of reach? If so, you are not alone. The 3-minute breathing space is a practice designed to help you bring mindfulness into those very moments. It's a bridge between the formal sitting and movement practices and your everyday life. It's one of the most important practices you'll learn in this course. Mothers in our groups tell us it's the practice they rely on the most.

How is it that 3 minutes can provide such benefit? We invite you to practice it now to give yourself a chance to explore this question based on your own experience.

Practice Now

Take a "3-minute breathing space" now. Take a few moments to get settled in your space, and then you can begin with the "3-Minute Breathing Space" audio (Track 10) to guide your practice.

Reflections on Practice

What did you notice in the first step? What was present in your thoughts, emotions, and body sensations?

_____

_____

_____

_____

What did you notice in the second step? What did you feel as you gathered your awareness with the breath?

_____

_____

_____

_____

What did you notice in the third step? What was present as you expanded your awareness to your full experience?

_____

_____

_____

_____

_____

As you reflect on your vision for staying well during pregnancy, postpartum, and beyond, how might this practice support you along the staying-well path?

_____

_____

_____

_____

_____

Circle of Mothers

"You know, my son didn't sleep very well. He slept really great when he was really small, and then at around 6 months he started sleeping poorly. And that was really challenging, because we had gotten used to him sleeping well. So I started using the 3-minute breathing when he would wake up in the night. As I was getting out of bed, I would take just those few minutes to notice what I was feeling—usually some mixture of heavy with sleep and irritated—and breathing for even just two or three breaths before I got to his crib. I noticed that I was more open to picking him up or getting a bottle or whatever it was he needed when I did the breathing space before."

"When I got pregnant, my daughter was 2 years old, and she was throwing temper tantrums. There were a couple of times where I could just feel myself getting overwhelmed and using that 3-minute breathing space. . . . I said, Okay, I'm going to go into the other room and do that practice. Normally, I would just get caught up in thinking 'What is wrong with this child? She's so strong-willed, she's going to end up in jail some day!' The 3-minute practice helps you stop yourself in your tracks when you start to kind of just get a little ahead of yourself and what's actually happening. I think some of the longer mindfulness practices were okay to use at the time, but I found myself using them less over time. The 3-minute breathing space is a keeper; it is really practical."

Daily Practice for Lesson 2

Practice the 3-minute breathing space every day.

◆ To make it a routine part of your day, choose three set times that you will practice it daily. This is such an important practice because it's brief and adaptable for so many moments of life; however, these very strengths also make it hard to remember. Even though it's only 3 minutes, it is easy to forget to do this practice as you're getting started. For this reason, women find it helpful to link these times to regular, daily events, such as waking up, arriving home at the end of the day, and going to bed. Take a moment now to write down the three times at which you will practice each day. Even with this advance planning, if you forget one practice time or even a whole day, you can always begin again!

Time #1: _____

Time #2: _____

Time #3: _____

You can use the audio guide to support your practice each time or just use it once a day to keep the instructions fresh in your mind. A written summary of the instructions is included with the homework for this session as a support for your practice when you choose not to use the audio track.

◆ Each time you practice, circle a "3MBS" (for 3-minute breathing space) on your weekly Practice Journal at the end of this chapter.

Lesson 3. Noticing in Daily Life

Being pregnant or a new mom provides you with nearly limitless opportunities to practice mindfulness through the daily activity of connecting with your baby. Our friend and colleague Nancy Bardacke, who teaches mindfulness to couples as they prepare for birthing and early parenting (*www.mindfulbirthing.org*), offered us the practice of "being with baby" to share with you. In this lesson, we provide two sets of guidance on "being with baby"—one for pregnancy and one for early parenting.

In this lesson, we acknowledge the reality that life can be hard while pregnant and parenting. Many of the moments of "being with baby" are sweet and enjoyable—but not all. Just like life in general, it's a mix of pleasant and unpleasant, easy and hard. For this reason, in this lesson, we build on the practice of noticing pleasant events, which we learned in the first class, while also being aware of unpleasant events as they are occurring.

Being with Baby

During Pregnancy

The experiences of pregnancy can be a great mindfulness teacher. There is great diversity in the ways that women experience pregnancy, and these experiences change with each week and trimester. Once you're in the second half of pregnancy, you begin to feel your baby move. At first you feel occasional little flutters—some people say the sensations feel like "tiny bubbles"—but these might not occur very often. As your baby grows bigger and stronger, the sensations change, and you feel them many times throughout the day. Sometimes you might feel a few quick little pokes. Other times you might experience dramatic, wave-like movements that momentarily change the shape of your entire belly. Or you might feel short, rhythmic pulsing (like what it feels like when the baby is having hiccups). These sensations from the baby's movements offer opportunities to practice mindfulness in daily life, which can connect you to the wonder of the experience of pregnancy itself and strengthen these critical skills for staying well. You can do the "being with baby" practice anytime you notice the baby moving (see the written instructions in the daily practice for this class, page 78). "Being with baby" during pregnancy is a way to practice being more awake and aware in your daily life before the baby is born. It's also excellent preparation for parenting.

If you're in the first half of pregnancy, remember that it's entirely normal not to feel movement from the baby. For some women, this time brings a comfortable sense of ease and connection to the baby, even without experiencing movement. For others, early pregnancy brings a world of discomfort, including nausea, exhaustion, and/or the sense that being pregnant is unfamiliar and strange. Some women with histories of depression or anxiety struggle with feeling connected to the baby or the idea of being pregnant at all. As Becca, a first-time mom reflected: "The ultrasounds help in making it feel more real, but most of the time I feel like I'm in limbo. I hope that with continued practice I can feel more connected to the tiny human growing inside of me. It's hard, though, because I keep thinking that it should feel more natural, but it really doesn't." Such experiences can be intensified for women who have struggled with infertility or have a history of pregnancy loss. Often, women can feel increased anxiety focusing on whether the baby is moving or not (or, for first-time moms, how to know if sensations are movement or something else). If any of these experiences are true for you, it's okay to set the "being with baby" practice aside and return to it later in your pregnancy or after the baby is born. In the meantime, continue to focus on mindfulness with other daily activities, such as drinking tea, showering, and eating.

During Early Parenting

If you are a new mother, you already know that your baby will "ask you" to stop, pay attention, and be present many times throughout your day and night, regardless of what you are doing at any particular moment. You can strengthen the skill of mindfulness by using the "being with baby" practice for new moms along with the "Being with Baby" audio (Track 11) or the "Feeding Baby" audio (Track 17).

As Audra described, these practices can be a tremendous support in adapting to the rhythms of early parenting: "One of the practices that has been most helpful to me is 'being with baby.' I practiced it a lot while I was pregnant. I would take a few minutes every time she moved to just put my hand on my belly and notice what she was doing. She was such an active one, it would go from flutters to earthquakes! I'm so glad I did that because it's really helped me since she was born. Sometimes I think that she will never sleep, and I do the 'being with baby' practice while I am rocking her or walking around with her at night. I notice the sensations of moving back and forth or side to side. I notice how she can go quickly from squirmy to tense to even little moments of relaxing. Paying attention to those movements helps me stay in the moment rather than get caught up in thinking that this will never end."

Pleasant and Unpleasant Events

In our second class, we focused on paying attention to pleasant events and invited you to take time to notice the specific elements of pleasant events. This practice reminds us that it's easy to miss the many small, pleasant moments in life without making a deliberate effort to pay attention to them. This practice also teaches the specific skill of identifying the particular elements of an experience. Identifying these elements can provide a lot of valuable information that gets lost when we stay at the general level. For example, imagine the difference between noticing "It was nice to see my friend after so many months" and noticing "I felt such a sense of lightness when I was with her and really happy. I noticed thinking that she is a really trustworthy person, and I can count on her, even when we haven't talked in a while."

In today's class, we expand our practice focus to include unpleasant events. In the same way that you noticed specific thoughts, feelings, and body sensations while having a pleasant experience, it's possible to notice them while having an unpleasant experience. Sometimes people report that they don't want to do this practice. They may think, "I don't want to pay attention to something unpleasant! I would like to avoid unpleasant things, not focus more on them." One of the core lessons of this course is that turning toward our experiences rather than ignoring them helps to provide valuable information. One of the first steps to dealing skillfully with unpleasant events is to simply be present with them. Over time, as we move into later classes, we also will focus on developing the skills to respond wisely and effectively to unpleasant events.

Daily Practice for Lesson 3

Practice mindfulness of routine experiences, including unpleasant ones, every day.

♦ Each day, practice mindfulness using your choice of a routine event or "being with baby" (using the written instructions if you are pregnant or the "Being with Baby" audio, Track 11, if you are a new mom). Notice and record in your Practice Journal any thoughts or feelings that arise as you do this practice.

♦ Each day, pay attention to one unpleasant experience, preferably while it's occurring. Remember, the unpleasant experience can be simple and brief, such as tasting an unappealing food or hearing a harsh noise, or it can be more complicated, such as having a challenging interaction with someone. Use the Unpleasant Experiences Practice Journal at the end of this chapter to record the components of your experience. Record thoughts as if you were speaking them out loud, in the words that actually came to your mind, and describe emotions and body sensations in as much detail as possible.

Daily Practice Summary

To recap, we invite you to do the following daily practices and record your experiences in the Practice Journal below.

Lesson 1

• On days 1, 3, 5, and 7, do a sitting practice. Practice with 25 minutes of mindful breathing, using Track 8 for the "25-Minute Sitting Meditation" practice (or, on very busy days, Track 7 for the "10-Minute Breathing Meditation" practice).

• On days 2, 4 and 6, do a movement practice. If you select the yoga practice, use the "25-Minute Yoga Practice" (Video 3), or, on especially busy days, the "10-Minute Yoga Practice" (Video 2). If you select the walking practice, listen and practice along with the 8-minute "Walking Meditation" instructions (Track 9).

• Briefly record in your Practice Journal the sensations, thoughts, or emotions that you notice.

Lesson 2

- Practice using the "3-minute breathing space" three times a day, at set times that you have decided in advance, and record the number of times you practice in your Practice Journal. You may use the guided instructions ("3-Minute Breathing Space"/Track 10) or the brief "reminder" instructions below once you have practiced with the audio guidance a few times.

3-Minute Breathing Space Instructions

The first thing we do with this practice, because it is brief, is to take an intentional posture that is both relaxed and alert. Allow your posture, whether sitting or standing, to express a sense of being present, at ease, and awake. You may close your eyes if it feels comfortable for you. The 3-minute breathing space involves three steps; take about 1 minute to practice each of the steps.

Step 1. Becoming Aware

Ask yourself, What am I experiencing right now? What thoughts are present in my mind? What emotions are present? Briefly scanning the body, ask what sensations are present. Allow whatever is present in your experience to be, pleasant or unpleasant. Simply ask, What is my experience right now?

Step 2. Gathering

Gather your awareness to focus on the sensations of breathing at the belly. Focus on the movement, moment by moment, breath by breath, as best you can. Feel when the breath is moving in and when the breath is moving out. Just bring your awareness, again and again, to the pattern of movement at the belly. Gathering yourself, use the anchor of the breath to be present.

Step 3. Expanding

Now, as a third step, allow awareness to expand. As well as being aware of the breath, include a sense of the body as a whole in your awareness. Allowing awareness to be more spacious, hold your full experience in this expanded awareness.

Then, when you're ready, allow your eyes to open. And as best you can, bring this expanded, more spacious, accepting awareness to the next moments of your day.

Lesson 3

- Practice noticing in daily life: either pay attention to a routine event, such as brushing your teeth, or do the "being with baby" practice. If you're pregnant and having physical sensations of the baby's movement, you can use the written instructions below. If you're early in pregnancy and don't yet experience many physical sensations, you can return to this section and begin this practice in the future. If you have a baby, you can use the "Being with Baby" audio (Track 11) to support your daily practice of "being with baby." Record your thoughts and feelings with your mindfulness of daily activity or "being with baby" practice in your Practice Journal.

- Notice and record the components of one unpleasant event each day in your Unpleasant Experiences Practice Journal.

Circle of Support

- On at least one day, talk with your support person about what you learned from this chapter and what you're noticing in your daily practices. Record any reflections based on these conversations in the Circle of Support Reflections.

- If you practice "being with baby," you might consider sharing the experience with your support person this week. Doing so allows your support person to be more connected with you during your pregnancy or during the postpartum. You might find that it increases your sense of wonder and enjoyment to share the experience with someone who cares for you.

"Being with Baby" Practice during Pregnancy Instructions

Let the sensations of the baby moving be a reminder to bring your attention fully to your body in the present moment. If you are in a situation where you can close your eyes while you are paying attention, experiment with that.

Drop down into just being pregnant in this moment, feel the sensations, and know you are feeling them.

As you pay attention to the sensations, see if you can also be aware of your breath in the belly, aware of the rising of the belly on the inhalation and the falling of the belly on the exhalation. You may want to bring your hand to your belly, feeling both the baby's movements and the movements from your breath under your hand.

If, or more likely when, your mind wanders, bring it back to the sensations of your hand on your belly and the movements of the breath and the baby beneath your hand. Notice any thoughts and/or feelings that arise as you do this. Practice "being with baby" for as long as is practical.

- During pregnancy, ask your support person to read the instructions and then gently bring a hand to your belly and focus attention on the sensations from the baby's movements. You can bring your awareness to the point of contact between the person's hand and your belly, perhaps noticing sensations of warmth or pressure, as well as noticing the sensations caused by the movements of the baby within.

- During the postpartum, you may ask your support person to listen and practice along with you to the instructions on Track 11. Do this quietly together, without speaking, for several minutes. Share your experience with each other, if you care to, when the practice is completed.

Practice Journal

	Day 1	Day 2	Day 3
Lesson 1 Practice Reflections: What did you notice in your sitting or movement practice today? Remember to alternate between these two from day to day.			
Example: *I moved locations today, from the couch to the exercise ball. I enjoyed the ability to sway a bit when I felt tightness in my back. I noticed hearing birds right outside of my window at the start of the practice, and I noticed smiling.*			
Lesson 2 Practice Reflections: 3-minute breathing space (3MBS). Please circle each time you do one of your three daily 3MBS practices.			
	3MBS 3MBS 3MBS	3MBS 3MBS 3MBS	3MBS 3MBS 3MBS
Lesson 3 Practice Reflections: Record here any thoughts or feelings you notice in your mindfulness of daily activity or your "being with baby" practice.			
Example: *Yikes! I completely forgot! I am going to put a sticky note on the tea kettle to remind myself in the morning.*			

Practice Journal

Day 4	Day 5	Day 6	Day 7
3MBS	3MBS	3MBS	3MBS
3MBS	3MBS	3MBS	3MBS
3MBS	3MBS	3MBS	3MBS

Unpleasant Experiences Practice Journal

	Day 1	Day 2	Day 3
What was the experience?			
Example: *Waiting for my friend to call me back after leaving two messages for her about taking care of my 2-year-old while I go to the doctor. Realizing it's late and she won't call tonight.*			
What sensations in your body were present during the experience?			
Example: *Tightness in the pit of my stomach, heaviness in my chest.*			
What moods or feelings were present during the experience?			
Example: *Hurt, disappointed, worried.*			
What thoughts were present during the experience?			
Example: *"Why is she ignoring me?" "Did I do something to make her mad?" "I really need to know if she can help." "What am I going to do if she can't help?"*			
What thoughts are in your mind now as you write this down?			
Example: *I hadn't realized how much this was bothering me.*			

Unpleasant Experiences Practice Journal

Day 4	Day 5	Day 6	Day 7

Circle of Support Reflections

What did you notice in connecting with your support person this week?

CLASS 4

Opening to Difficulty and Uncertainty

Where there is no struggle, there is no strength.
—Oprah Winfrey

This chapter focuses on three key lessons:

1. **The mindfulness skills you've already developed can help you open to difficulty and uncertainty, which are frequent aspects of the experience of pregnancy and early parenting.** We help you expand the foundation of mindfulness practice you have been building to respond skillfully to difficulty and uncertainty.

2. **The 3-minute breathing space is a wonderful tool to help you cope with moments of difficulty and uncertainty. It is always available to you!** We invite you to integrate this practice when responding to difficulty and uncertainty in your daily life.

3. **It is possible and important to recognize the signs of entering the territory of depression and anxiety during pregnancy and early parenting.** We help you understand these signs and identify the ones that are most informative for you.

Lesson 1. Opening to Difficulty and Uncertainty

Opening to Difficulty

Pregnancy and postpartum are no strangers to difficult times. Common challenges include adjusting to the changes in your body, worrying about finances, making sure you are eating well, and getting enough sleep. As one mom commented, "It feels like taking care of a pregnant body is a full-time job. I get exhausted thinking about all the things I should be doing every day. And I don't think I've ever gotten all that protein." The difficulties of pregnancy shift once the baby is born, and yet other new challenges frequently arise. The ups and downs of tensions in your relationships, the demands of caring for a new baby, keeping up a household, and attending to the needs of other children or a job are common difficulties. If your baby is born early, has health problems, or your birth experience is traumatic, you may enter a world of entirely new difficulties. Other major life stressors, like moving, losing a job, or the illness or death of a relative, may feel more familiar but have an unfamiliar impact as you are also coping with caring for a new baby. Even minor events, like a long line in the grocery store, can be experienced as difficult. Given this context of difficulty, what makes the difference between maintaining your well-being and getting overwhelmed or beginning to slide back into depression? *How* you respond to such difficulties can make an important difference.

Responding to Difficulty

What do we mean when we say "respond to" difficulties?

Think of a difficulty in your life right now that is related to being pregnant or caring for a new baby. Select one that is important to you but is not the most difficult thing you can imagine. Perhaps consider a situation that is about a 3 on a difficulty scale of 0 (not difficult at all) to 10 (the most difficult ever). Ask yourself, when facing this difficulty:

- Do you *strive or reach for* particular thoughts, memories, emotions, or sensations?
- Do you *avoid or push away* particular thoughts, memories, emotions, or sensations?
- Do you *dwell on or get stuck* in particular thoughts, memories, emotions, or sensations?

If these questions feel abstract to you, perhaps consider the experiences of Andrea. She identified difficulty sleeping as an important concern for her, and in reflecting on how she responds to this difficulty, she discovered that she responded in each of these ways at different times.

When experiencing discomfort in her body at night, particularly tension in her lower back, she discovered that she tossed and turned, seeking the kind of physical comfort she recalled feeling in bed before becoming pregnant. She wanted so much to feel free from that aching and burning in her lower back.

She also realized that she frequently sought to push away the discomfort and sleeplessness. She would tell herself, with a twinge of frustration and panic in the middle of the night, "Just ignore it and go to sleep!"

Finally, she also got stuck on the difficulty of sleeplessness. In the middle of the afternoon, when her energy was particularly low, she would review, again and again, her lack of a good night's sleep and her frustration toward the sensations of discomfort. She found herself thinking, repeatedly: "How am I going to get through 20 more weeks of this if I can't get a good night's sleep? How will I deal with everything I have to take care of now, and what about when the baby comes? Will I ever sleep again?"

These are three common responses to difficulty that actually can make life harder and increase vulnerability to feeling down, stressed, or overwhelmed. This can be particularly so when facing situations or emotions that are not wanted, expected, or controlled—as is often the case during pregnancy and early parenting.

An important lesson from this class is that the most effective way to care for yourself is to act on the basis of opening to what is present, even if it's difficult.

Awareness of what you're experiencing—even when it's painful, scary, frustrating, and hard—gives you the chance to act with greater wisdom and balance. Instead of reacting on automatic pilot, you may respond more skillfully to what's happening, even if it is most decidedly not what you want, by recognizing and opening to your thoughts, feelings, and body sensations.

You may have had moments in your daily practice following our last class in which you noticed unpleasant experiences during the yoga or sitting meditation practices or in your daily life activities. These unpleasant experiences can offer valuable opportunities to notice how you respond to difficulty and to practice new ways of responding. Perhaps, as for Andrea, the difficulties are physical, like an aching back. Or perhaps the difficulty is a particular emotion that arises or a thought about a situation or experience in your life. Let's explore how you respond to difficulty through paying attention to unpleasant experiences that arise during a practice right now.

Practice Now

When you're ready, please do 10 minutes of mindful yoga (use Video 2). Then continue with a 10-minute sitting meditation (using audio Track 7, "10-Minute Breathing Meditation"). When you're finished, please return to reflect on your experience.

Reflections on Practice

What did you notice while doing the yoga and sitting practices?

_____

_____

_____

_____

"When I was doing the yoga, I felt a little wobbly. It was a pleasure to be moving, but there was so much tension in my body. When I was sitting, I was aware of how tight and taut my belly feels. It's hard to get a full breath. And I was thinking a lot about work. I kept wanting to stop the practice to return a phone call. It was stressing me out that I wasn't just taking care of it, and I felt a little frantic just sitting."

Did you notice yourself responding to particular thoughts, memories, emotions, or sensations that arose during the yoga or sitting practices in any of these ways—striving or reaching, avoiding or pushing away, dwelling on or getting stuck?

_____

_____

_____

_____

_____

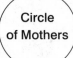

"When I was doing the yoga, I definitely was striving to feel relaxed. I wanted to get rid of all of that tension as I moved with the instructions. It didn't really happen, and the more I wanted to feel relaxed, the less relaxed I felt! When I was doing the sitting practice, I brought my attention back to breathing when I was thinking about that phone call. So I would notice 'not breath' and then come back to feeling my breathing, but it was like needing to make the phone call was in the background all the time and I just wanted it to go away. I wanted to push away the tension and the phone call, and the more strongly I pushed, the more they seemed to be all I was noticing. Ironic and irritating!"

As you reflect on your vision for staying well during pregnancy, postpartum, and beyond, how might awareness of the ways in which we can strive for, avoid or push away, or dwell on particular states support you along the staying-well path?

_____

_____

_____

_____

_____

Circle of Mothers

"Wow, this was challenging. It's hard for me to just be aware of tension, stress, and all of that without getting frustrated and wanting things to be different. It's like I'm in a battle with them, though I realize now that the battle is all happening within my own mind and body. If they are there, then they tend to take over. I push against them or get stuck in them. These ways of responding to difficulty don't actually help me. They keep me caught in this cycle of struggle. This practice helps me see the ways I'm repeating this cycle by how I am responding automatically, but it's really hard to respond differently once it gets started."

It Takes Practice

Many mothers struggle with opening to difficulty. If you experience even the idea of opening to difficulty as challenging, know that you're not alone!

Andrea, who experienced the difficulty of sleepless nights, said: "I really, really struggled with Lesson 1 this week. I felt a bit lost and unable to cope. I feel afraid about the impact of the tension that I feel on my baby, and doing the practice in Lesson 1 highlighted how much work I need to do with responding more effectively to difficulty, especially those that are not likely to go away anytime soon. I think such openness is a skill, and I don't have this skill yet."

Andrea is 100% correct in her realization that opening to difficulty is a skill and one that takes practice. It may be helpful to keep in mind the steps described in the acronym OPEN to help support you in practicing the skill of opening.

> **Observe** *what* is most predominant in your moment-by-moment experience. Whatever it is, simply notice it.
>
> **Put a name** to *how* you are relating to what is predominant in your experience. Are you reacting in any of these ways:
>
> - Striving or reaching for experiences?
> - Avoiding or pushing away experiences?
> - Dwelling on or getting stuck in experiences?
>
> **Explore** how these automatic reactions can be the opposite of opening to what is present.
>
> **Now,** in just this moment, practice letting go of the effort to make things different than they are. Practice opening to what is right now, rather than trying to make things fit some idea of how things "should" be.

As with Andrea, opening to difficulty didn't come automatically or easily to Becca. She describes how she practiced with using the acronym OPEN to help respond wisely to difficulty at home. Becca found herself thinking frequently about the millions of things on her daily to-do list as she managed her household, kids, new baby, and work. She shared with us her experience of completing this lesson during a particularly challenging week. She described sitting in the kitchen, listening to the Drinking Tea Meditation recording. It was a simple practice that she intended to do each morning. This morning, however, her kids were screaming in the background, and her mind kept darting to everything she had to get done, including the mountain of dirty dishes in the sink, her kids being rowdy in the other room, and her worry that they would wake up the baby. Then she remembered the instructions to OPEN:

"First I **observed** what I was feeling. I can't say that part was pleasant. I observed that I was thinking a lot, worrying a lot, hearing the kids' noise. I observed my shoulders were so tight, they were up at about my ears! It felt like a tight block. When I exhaled, I kind of released some of the tension in my shoulders, and the tension sensation in my shoulders softened a bit.

"Then I **put a name on** how I was reacting. I asked myself: 'Am I striving for something here? Am I avoiding or pushing away? Am I dwelling or getting stuck?' I realized that I was pushing away a lot of my experiences. I was saying to myself, 'I hate this; I can't even get a few minutes of peace.' I just wanted it to all stop. I had the urge to give up, turn off the recording, and go get breakfast ready, or just yell at them—'Be quiet!'

"Next I **explored** how these reactions were the opposite of opening. Instead of allowing myself to experience what was happening, I was focused on my thoughts of how things should be, like I should be able to get a few minutes of peace and quiet to do the practice for this class, the kids should be able to occupy themselves for a few minutes, I should be more organized.

"Finally, I remembered the last part: **now.** Just for a few seconds, I practiced saying, 'It is what it is.' I did that for a few breaths, and I noticed that my exhales were a little deeper and smoother, like I was letting go. By this point, the recording had stopped, and I just sat there for a few breaths. The noise around me hadn't gotten any quieter, but I was sitting there breathing in the midst of all of that noisiness. Unlike a few moments before, though, now I wasn't fighting it. That was a big difference! I opened myself to a new experience of relating to the stress and chaos around me, and it helped a lot with doing what needed to be done at that moment—protecting those few minutes in the morning for my practice. It allowed me to go into the other room and respond more calmly to the kids and then return to the kitchen to get them some breakfast and start in on the dishes."

As you practice in this way, like Becca, it's important to remember that opening to what is difficult is *not* a quick fix. It also is not resigning yourself to days of unwashed dishes, unruly children clamoring for your attention, and no time for yourself. Opening allows you to become fully aware of difficulties, and then, if appropriate, to *respond* in skillful ways rather than to *react* in knee-jerk fashion, with automatic, old (often unhelpful) strategies for dealing with difficulties.

Thus, just as Becca realized that she could practice with a sense of peace in the middle of her children's ruckus (rather than giving up her practice or yelling at them), you might discover new possibilities as you open to what you don't want or believe should be different.

Using the OPEN acronym can be a helpful support. We encourage you to practice with this acronym in your sitting and movement practice this week or, if it is relevant, in your daily practice times, such as Becca's experience of drinking tea mindfully. The difficulties you encounter may be events happening around you, like Becca's, or they may be internal, such as uncomfortable thoughts, emotions, and body sensations. They all provide a wonderful context for learning! Remember what Andrea said—"Openness is a skill"—and we encourage you to allow yourself to be a learner.

Opening to Uncertainty

Not all difficulties are created equal. For many women, uncertainty is one of the common difficulties that arise during pregnancy and early parenting, which causes a great deal of heartache and hardship. If there is one thing to "expect when you are expecting," it is the unexpected. If you are someone who tends to like having control or influence over what is happening within and around you, then this difficulty of pregnancy and early parenting may be particularly challenging. Every day is filled with one uncertainty or another, and a host of events over which you have little to no control arise on a frequent basis.

This context of uncertainty—and not being able to control it—can contribute to feeling down, stressed, or overwhelmed. Practicing opening to uncertainty specifically—in addition to other forms of difficulty—can be *helpful* in coping with this inherent aspect of pregnancy and the postpartum. That said, "helpful" does not mean "easy."

Renee expressed this realization with great honesty: "I was most challenged with opening to uncertainty this week. I didn't really feel prepared for this, like I was thrown into the deep end of a pool without knowing how to keep afloat or swim. It was helpful to remind myself of the OPEN acronym and tell myself, 'I'm just learning, it's okay to struggle, especially because these are big challenges!' I'm glad that I did the practices in Lesson 2 because they helped me realize how essential these skills are at this time in my life . . . and yet it *is* hard!"

One way to begin to practice with opening to uncertainty is to use your imagination to explore your responses to uncertain situations. Doing so is like wading into the shallow end of the pool because it's imaginal . . . rather than being faced with the actual situation. It can help you become familiar with your automatic responses to types of uncertainty that are relevant to being pregnant, giving birth, or your baby. This practice has been helpful for many women in strengthening the skill of opening to uncertainty. At the same time, it also can elicit strong emotion. Go slowly with the lessons of this week and allow yourself to pace your practice in a way that is most helpful for you. Take small steps into the shallow end of the pool. Know also that you can get out or rest on the side at any point and get back in when you're ready.

Practice Now

To begin with the uncertainty practice, we ask you to think of a number between 1 and 5. We'll explain in a bit how you'll use this number, but for now, just randomly pick one number between 1 and 5 and write it down here.

What is your number? ____

Next, reflect on some of your main preferences for the three periods of pregnancy, labor, and the postpartum. Listed below are some of the things that women often tell us are important to them. This list is not exhaustive, and there may be other dimensions that are important to you. Think about what matters most to *you* in terms of how things will go and what you want most.

- Vaginal birth versus C-section
- Normal prenatal test results versus results indicating concern with the baby
- Going full term (or post) versus induction
- No pain medication versus epidural
- Hospital birth versus other (home or birthing center)
- Episiotomy versus natural tearing
- Limit on people in the birthing room versus having everyone you choose
- Immediate skin-to-skin contact with baby versus baby taken to warming table
- Frequent fetal monitoring versus no to little fetal monitoring
- Healthy baby versus baby with special needs
- Breast feeding versus bottle feeding
- Baby that sleeps through most of the night versus up several times a night
- Easy-to-soothe baby versus fussy/colicky baby
- Lots of family/friends' input/advice versus little input/advice
- Planned date nights with partner versus spontaneous connections
- Father of baby more versus less involved with early parenting
- Other relatives or caregivers more versus less involved with baby

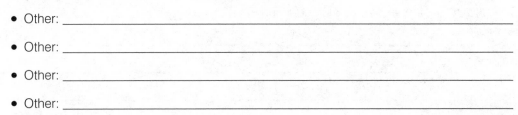

- Working outside the home versus being full-time mom
- Returning to work before versus after 12 weeks postpartum
- Other: _____
- Other: _____
- Other: _____
- Other: _____

Considering the list above and any that you may have added, write one item on each line below that describes how you *really* want things to go for you over the rest of your pregnancy, with labor and delivery, and after the baby is born.

1. _____
2. _____
3. _____
4. _____
5. _____

Read over your list above and reflect on how much you wish those things to be true for your experience during pregnancy, labor and delivery, and the postpartum.

Next, recalling the number that you selected above, write here the preference that corresponds to that number. Thus, if "4" was the number that you randomly selected above, here you would write the fourth item from your list of five.

What is the item associated with your number?

_____

Now imagine that this preference may not happen.

Perhaps close your eyes and imagine that, although you want this very much, it's not something you can count on or know for sure will occur. Even though the other four things may occur, in your imagination, practice opening to the possibility that this one preference may not come to be. Open to the possibility that it just may not happen.

In doing this practice, you are opening to the reality that despite your best intentions and desires, you cannot control all aspects of being pregnant, giving birth, or caring for a child. Take a moment to reflect on the thoughts, feelings, and body sensations that were present as you practiced letting go and opening to the uncertainty.

Reflections on Practice

What thoughts, feelings, and sensations in your body were present as you imagined that this thing you wanted very much did not occur?

_____

_____

_____

_____

_____

Circle of Mothers

"I immediately sought to push the thought that this might not happen out of my mind. No way!! I didn't even want to consider the prospect that my son might not be healthy in some way. In my head, I realize that it isn't something I can control entirely. Kids get sick and so do little babies. But, in the moment, I just thought, no way!"

"I didn't have a strong response when imagining this because I happened to pick a number for something that I want to happen, but I'm actually okay if it doesn't too. It was interesting, though, because I felt such strong relief that I hadn't picked number 1 because I think that would have been really hard to imagine!!"

*In what ways did you notice **avoiding or pushing away** the context of uncertainty and **striving or reaching** for greater control?*

_____

_____

_____

_____

_____

Circle of Mothers

"I actually put the workbook down at the end of the imaginal exercise. I literally wanted to push it away. I put my pen down defiantly. Forget it, I thought."

"I felt kind of relieved at first, but then I noticed that I was pushing away the possibility of not having the experiences that I identified with other numbers."

As you reflect on your vision for staying well during pregnancy, postpartum, and beyond, how might this practice of opening to uncertainty support you along the staying-well path?

_____

_____

_____

_____

_____

Circle of Mothers

"I prefer to have control or at least to influence what happens. This practice felt like a lot more than dipping my toe into the shallow end of the pool. I don't even like imagining the unknown and especially about something that matters as much to me as my baby's health. He's so little and vulnerable, and I want to control everything possible. At the same time, I know it's the truth. I want to have more ease in the presence of the unknown as I learn how to be his mom. I want to allow him to explore and discover and grow without my always being tense about the unknown. As much as it is hard for me, doing this practice is helping me develop the flexibility and greater ease that is so important to me. I resist this practice in particular, but I do it for both him and me."

"As much as I don't want to admit it, I cannot control the future. Pregnancy has made me come up against this concept time and time again. Even if it's just an illusion, holding on to the possibility of control helps me feel safe and comfortable. The unknown scares the heck out of me, especially as I stare down this final trimester to giving birth. I don't love this opening to uncertainty practice, but I definitely see its value."

Daily Practice for Lesson 1

Do a practice each day, alternating between the sitting practice and the yoga or walking movement practice. You may select either the yoga or walking practice on the movement day, or you may do both on each of those days. As you practice, allow moments of difficulty and uncertainty to arise naturally. When they do, use the OPEN acronym to strengthen your skills of opening to difficulty and uncertainty.

◆ Sitting meditation: days 1, 3, 5, and 7. Practice with 25 minutes of mindful breathing. If you like, you may begin by reviewing the "Introduction to

Sitting Meditation" (Track 6) and then use the audio recording for the "25-Minute Sitting Meditation" practice (Track 8) to guide your practice. On days in which it is challenging to make time for the 25-minute practice, the "10-Minute Breathing Meditation" practice may be a helpful option (Track 7).

♦ Yoga or walking practice: days 2, 4 and 6. If you select the yoga, practice along with the "25-Minute Yoga Practice" (Video 3), or on especially busy days you might rely on the "10-Minute Yoga Practice" (Video 2). If you select the walking, please listen and practice along with the 8-minute mindful "Walking Meditation" instructions (Track 9). You can do the walking practice indoors or out, although it may be easier to practice indoors the first few times.

♦ Briefly record in your Practice Journal the sensations, thoughts, or emotions that you notice each time you practice. Note any times and observations about working with the OPEN steps.

Lesson 2. Relying on the 3-Minute Breathing Space to Cope with Difficulty and Uncertainty

The 3-minute breathing space can be a wonderful support in the moments in which life goes in unexpected or difficult ways. You have been making the 3-minute breathing space a routine daily practice over the last week, and now we can build on this foundation by bringing the 3-minute breathing space to coping with difficult moments and uncertainty, such as we have been exploring. It provides a way to step out of automatic pilot reactions of reaching, pushing away, or dwelling and allows us to open to the unknown, uncertain, and undesired with greater ease.

Elena reflected on her experience with the 3-minute breathing space during difficult moments: "The three 3-minute breathing spaces helped me calm down a couple times this week, when things felt like they were becoming too overwhelming or stressful. I'm not sure if it is the pregnancy or not, but I find myself more irritable than usual for me. The three 3-minute breathing spaces helped me cope with that irritability and not let it spiral into doing or saying something I might later regret."

As a reminder, here are the steps of the 3-minute breathing space, which you can extend for coping with difficult times. You may find it helpful to read over these instructions fully before you practice, or you can read over these and then listen to the recording on audio Track 10, "Three 3-Minute Breathing Spaces," as you practice.

Take an intentional posture that is both relaxed and dignified. Allow your posture, whether sitting or standing, to express a sense of being present, at ease, and awake. You may close your eyes if it feels comfortable for you.

In Step 1, ask yourself, What am I experiencing right now? What thoughts are present in my mind? What emotions are present? Briefly scanning the body, ask what sensations are present. Allow whatever is present in your experience to be, pleasant or unpleasant. Simply ask, What is my experience right now?

In Step 2, gather your awareness to focus on the sensations of breathing at the belly. Focus on the movement, moment by moment, breath by breath, as best you can, knowing when the breath is moving in and when the breath is moving out. Bring your awareness again and again to the pattern of movement at the belly. Gathering yourself, use the anchor of the breath to be present.

In Step 3, allow awareness to expand. As well as being aware of the breath, include a sense of the body as a whole in your awareness. Allowing awareness to be more spacious, hold your full experience in this expanded awareness.

When you're ready, open your eyes, bringing this expanded, more spacious, accepting awareness to the next moments of your day.

Practice Now

Now bring something to mind that is difficult—although not the most difficult thing you can imagine. Perhaps consider a situation that is about a 3 on a difficulty scale of 0 (not difficult at all) to 10 (the most difficult ever).

Practice the steps described above, supported by listening to Track 10, as you bring to mind this level-3 difficulty. When you're finished, please return to reflect on your experience.

Reflections on Practice

What did you notice in your thoughts, emotions, and body sensations as you brought the area of difficulty to mind (Step 1)?

_____

_____

_____

_____

What did you notice in the second step? What did you feel as you gathered your awareness at the breath?

_____

_____

_____

_____

What did you notice in the third step? What was present as you expanded your awareness to your full experience in the context of the difficulty?

_____

_____

_____

_____

As you reflect on your vision for staying well during pregnancy, postpartum, and beyond, how might this practice support you along the staying-well path?

_____

_____

_____

_____

Circle of Mothers

"There are times when I get snippy and I can feel my shoulders tensing up, like when I'm feeling rushed and I can't go as fast as I did before I was pregnant. I was walking with my husband and some friends from the parking garage to the restaurant. I just tried to power through it and keep up with them. But when I got to the restaurant, I was exhausted and tense and stressed. On the way back, I paused and slowed down and used that little 3-minute breathing space when I noticed I was starting to feel anxious about keeping up. I noticed how tense in my shoulders and neck I was and all my thoughts and emotions, then I took a few breaths, and I found I could keep going, just a little slower than the others. I laughed to myself and the baby because it didn't even bother me in that moment that they all seemed clueless about us needing more time."

"I use it when I'm nursing the baby, and I feel discouraged because it's been really hard to get her to latch. So, when I do the second step and take those deep breaths and I expand, I can just notice holding her hand or rubbing her head and that sort of thing, rather than being all caught up in thinking that I can't do this."

"When I put my son in his play pen when I need to get something done during the day, and he just howls, I walk away, and often I just grit my teeth and think about how I am going to get through this and how I can't get a moment to get anything done. Now I use the 3-minute breathing space right there. It is one of the most helpful coping tools that I've learned. It's a really good time to do that. I find a way to breathe."

It takes practice to make the 3-minute breathing space available during difficult times. We invite you to take additional breathing spaces when you're experiencing difficulty. These difficult times might include feeling tension in the body, experiencing challenging specific emotions (e.g., irritation, guilt, fear, embarrassment), a general sense of being overwhelmed or stressed, or that sinking feeling when you realize that things are not going as you thought they would. The goal of the breathing space at such times is not to make the difficulty or uncertainty "go away" but rather to support you in responding to what you're experiencing with greater ease and balance.

Daily Practice for Lesson 2

Practice the 3-minute breathing space every day.

◆ To support you in accessing the 3-minute breathing space during difficult times, we invite you to begin the practice of taking additional breathing spaces when you're experiencing difficulty. Even though it's only 3 minutes, it's easy to forget to do this practice as you're getting started; thus, keeping up your routine 3-minute breathing space practice is important too and will make it easier to rely on the breathing space during difficult times. Reaffirm here that you will do your routine breathing spaces at the following times each day.

Time #1: _____

Time #2: _____

Time #3: _____

You can use the audio guidance of Track 10, "3-Minute Breathing Space," to support your practice each time or just use it once a day to keep the instructions fresh in your mind. In your Practice Journal at the end of this chapter, circle a "3MBS" (for 3-minute breathing space) for each time you complete the routine daily practice and "Coping 3MBS" for each use of the breathing space during difficult times.

Lesson 3. It Is Possible and Important to Recognize the Signs of Entering the Territory of Depression and Anxiety during Pregnancy and Parenting

Although people often assume that being pregnant and being a new mom are the happiest times of a woman's life, such assumptions do not fit with the day-to-day experiences of many women. As you are now undoubtedly well aware, there are many difficulties and uncertainties that cause stress and challenge during pregnancy and parenting.

In fact, rates of depression during these times are no different than at other times in a woman's life. Ten to 15% of women meet diagnostic criteria for what mental health professionals call "major depression" during the first year following the birth of a child, and major depression during pregnancy is equally common. An even larger group of women experience symptoms of depression that get in the way of living their daily lives or cause distress, even if such symptoms don't cross the threshold for "major depression."

Moreover, depression has many close cousins, such as anxiety and stress, that commonly occur among pregnant and postpartum women. For women who have been depressed in the past, the rates of depression during pregnancy and postpartum are higher than among those women who have not been depressed previously in their lives.

Despite the high rates of depression and anxiety, the tools of this class can help you reduce symptoms of depression and prevent relapse into major depression during pregnancy and the postpartum, even if you have a history of depression or current struggles with depressive or anxious symptoms.

Part of staying well is being aware of the territory of depression and anxiety during pregnancy and early parenting. Let's explore ways in which you might already be familiar with some parts of this territory. Listed below are various thoughts that pop into people's heads (thanks and credit to Steven D. Hollon for providing this list). Please read each thought and circle the ones that are familiar to you, the ones that tend to play most frequently or loudly during times when you're feeling down, stressed, or overwhelmed.

1. I feel like I'm up against the world.

2. I'm no good.

3. Why can't I ever succeed?

4. No one understands me.

5. I've let people down.

6. I don't think I can go on.

7. I wish I were a better person.

8. I'm so weak.

9. My life's not going the way I want it to.

10. I'm so disappointed in myself.

11. Nothing feels good anymore.

12. I can't stand this anymore.

13. I can't get started.

14. What's wrong with me?

15. I wish I were somewhere else.

16. I can't get things together.

17. I hate myself.

18. I'm worthless.

19. I wish I could just disappear.

20. What's the matter with me?

21. I'm a loser.

22. My life is a mess.

23. I'm a failure.

24. I'll never make it.

25. I feel so helpless.

26. Something has to change.

27. There must be something wrong with me.

28. My future is bleak.

29. It's just not worth it.

30. I can't finish anything.

Also consider another list of thoughts that often pop into women's heads during pregnancy. Please read each thought and circle the ones that are familiar to you, the ones that tend to play most frequently or loudly during times when you're feeling down, stressed, or overwhelmed.

1. I'm worried about the pain of contractions and the pain during delivery.

2. I'm anxious about the delivery because I've never experienced one before.

3. I'm worried about not being able to control myself during labor and fear that I'll scream.

4. I'm afraid our baby will be stillborn or will die during or immediately after delivery.

5. I'm afraid that our baby will suffer from a physical defect or worry that something will be physically wrong with the baby.

6. I sometimes think that our child will be in poor health or will be prone to illnesses.

7. I'm worried about not regaining my figure after delivery.

8. I'm worried that I'm unattractive.

9. I'm worried about how to cope when my baby is hard to soothe.

10. I'm worried about whether I will be a good mother.

11. I'm worried about whether I might do something to harm my baby, intentionally or unintentionally.

12. I'm worried about finances.

13. I'm worried about being a stay-at-home mom.

14. I'm worried about balancing my work and home life.

15. I'm worried about whether my relationship with my partner/husband will be challenged.

16. I'm worried that I won't do a good job as a new mom.

17. I'm worried that my baby won't love me.

18. I'm worried that I won't love my baby.

19. I'm worried that I won't know what to do as a new mom.

20. I'm worried that I won't be able to help my baby in the way that he or she will need.

21. I'm worried about not getting enough sleep.

22. I'm worried about physical intimacy with my partner/husband.

23. I'm worried about discomforts of pregnancy (such as heartburn, incontinence, back pain).

24. I'm worried about my weight.

25. I'm worried about body changes due to pregnancy and labor/delivery.

Now take a moment to review the thoughts that you circled across both lists and write below the "Top 10" that tend to play most often or loudly in your mind. Perhaps think of this activity like writing down the titles of the songs on your depression or anxiety playlist. If you have other "song titles" that play on your "Top 10" list that were not included on either of the two lists, write them in here as well.

1. _____

2. _____

3. _____

4. _____

5. _____

6. _____

7. _____

8. _____

9. _____

10. _____

Once you've listed them, take a moment to circle the number(s) next to the thoughts that are most troubling. Often, these are the thoughts that can hijack your attention and that you believe automatically, without even thinking to question them. When they are playing, you may believe that the thought is absolutely true. Also, these are the thoughts that you tend to get stuck in and dwell on or, conversely, the thoughts that you work hardest to push away.

Take a moment to reflect on the responses below from the circle of mothers as they reflect on the thoughts from their "Top 10" lists that are most troubling.

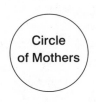

Circle of Mothers

"Number 14 on the first list is a big one for me. I think, 'What's wrong with me?' And also number 27. So I circled both of those—What's wrong with me? and There must be something wrong with me—because I just think that's my natural train of thought. I hate to admit it, but it is. That thought is kind of always there."

"Number 23 comes up a lot. It pops in even when things don't seem like that big a deal. Like this weekend, I thought the baby was coming, but when I went to the doctor I wasn't really even dilated and that was my first thought: I shouldn't have made such a big deal about it. I can't even tell if I'm going into labor. I'm a failure. And then I thought number 5 too, which comes up a lot, because I had my husband get out of work early to come to the doctor, so I thought I really let him down too with such a false alarm."

"I added one. I didn't see it on the list, so I added 'I'm always worried about the future.'"

> "Yeah, that's true for me too. I don't feel depressed. I think there was only one time in my life where I was really depressed. I think that on a general level I've always been a worrier, so anxiousness is probably more present, so on the second list I circled almost all of them!"

> "I try to fix everybody's problems at once, so it is kind of like numbers 10, 14, 15, and those kinds of thoughts on the second list, and then it gets so overwhelming I think sometimes I wish I could just disappear. So, I guess that's when number 19 on the first list jumps in."

You may have noticed some of your own "Top 10" showing up in the comments among the circle of mothers. Often women are surprised to learn that a thought that seemed so absolutely true of themselves (and about which they felt some shame or reluctance to share) is experienced by not just one but many other women in the circle. Over time, they realize that these thoughts are less about each individual woman than they are about the territory of depression, anxiety, and worry. By becoming familiar with this territory, you can begin to see that you are not alone and that the thoughts are less about you personally, less categorically true, and more about the nature of depression and anxiety. As a result, you may begin to feel less alone and begin to be more gentle with yourself for the ways you think and feel.

Susan described an experience in which recognizing the thoughts as part of her "Top 10" allowed her to respond in a new way:

> "Sometimes it's hard to know exactly what those thoughts are or to identify when they're playing because they're so automatic that I don't even notice that they've been playing in the background of my mind for a while. I noticed something last week when I was at a party for my nephew. I was a little tired, and I just didn't feel very social. I wasn't in a bad mood, but I knew that my husband hadn't been very eager to come, and so I was concerned that he wasn't enjoying himself. Plus, we had made such efforts to get a babysitter who could stay with the kids and take care of a 4-month-old; it's not so easy to find!
>
> "Then my mother-in-law commented on the fact that I didn't seem like I was having very much fun. Immediately, the thoughts started: Why can't I enjoy myself? Why do I have to worry about other people all the time? What's wrong with me that I'm so tired? I thought, everyone else seems to be having a better time—what's the matter with me? How can I not be enjoying myself when we hardly ever get to go out anymore and we're paying someone like $80 for this night!
>
> "It was like all of my "Top 10" kind of came in this quick series, like within 30 seconds. I started to feel awful. Then I was like, wait a minute, this is my "Top 10"! There are those familiar thoughts again. I don't have to dwell on them by asking myself why this and why that. I don't have to believe them. I don't have to argue with myself about them. I don't have to slide down that slippery slope to thinking what a horrible person, wife, and mother I am. I realized I can be just like I am; I do feel concerned about my husband, and that's okay. I

do feel concerned about the money for the babysitter, and that's okay. I feel tired tonight, and I'm just going to give myself a break.

"It was amazing how quickly one little comment from my mother-in-law just made me jump right into that whole thought process. I thought it was great that I noticed it."

Being aware of your "Top 10" thoughts can be helpful in responding in new ways in the moment. Being aware of the "Top 10" also can be useful in recognizing when you are becoming vulnerable to depression returning or to levels of stress or anxiety increasing to a point that gets in the way of your functioning well. An increase in the frequency or intensity of these types of thoughts (or the strength in which you believe them) can be like a signpost that you are entering the territory of depression or anxiety. But thoughts are not the only signposts. In addition to the thoughts, the territory of depression and anxiety include signs in the body and in your behavior. It's helpful to recognize these in general and also to identify ones that have been present for you in the past. Doing so can help you be more informed, aware, and able to take action early if you're starting to travel into the territory of depression and anxiety.

How can you know the difference between the normal changes of pregnancy and postpartum, including "the blues," and entering the territory of depression and anxiety?

Recognizing the Territory of Depression and Anxiety in the Midst of the Changes of Pregnancy and Parenting

During your pregnancy you'll experience a huge number of changes. Your body is changing, your relationships are changing, and you're preparing for all the changes that will come when your baby is born. It's common to feel tired and to experience disruptions in appetite and sleep during pregnancy. These experiences also can be symptoms of depression.

During the first few weeks after the baby is born, women can experience even more change. Adjusting to the new baby's rhythms and routines and learning how to feed and care for the baby can be challenging. Women's relationships with partners, family, and friends also undergo big changes. The majority of women experience the baby blues after giving birth. Women may feel sad and lonely, cry for no reason, and feel not like themselves. They may feel overwhelmed, anxious, or restless. They also may feel impatient or irritable. Women also may experience quickly going from feeling very happy to feeling very sad. If you feel this way, you are not alone.

There are a few ways that mental health professionals determine when changes in how a person is feeling indicate depression. Depression affects multiple aspects of a woman's life, including her body, emotions, thoughts, and ability to carry out everyday activities. These are the areas that mental health professionals pay attention to in determining whether a woman is experiencing concerning symptoms of depression. The Patient Health Questionnaire, or the "PHQ-9," on the next page is one of the common methods that mental health professionals use in working with women, and it's a very helpful way to learn more about the territory of depression.

Patient Health Questionnaire–9

	Not at all	Several days	More than half the days	Nearly every day
1. Little interest or pleasure in doing things	0	1	2	3
2. Feeling down, depressed, or hopeless	0	1	2	3
3. Trouble falling or staying asleep, or sleeping too much	0	1	2	3
4. Feeling tired or having little energy	0	1	2	3
5. Poor appetite or overeating	0	1	2	3
6. Feeling bad about yourself—or that you are a failure or have let yourself or your family down	0	1	2	3
7. Trouble concentrating on things, such as reading the newspaper or watching television	0	1	2	3
8. Moving or speaking so slowly that other people could have noticed. Or the opposite—being so fidgety or restless that you have been moving around a lot more than usual	0	1	2	3
9. Thoughts that you would be better off dead, or of hurting yourself in some way	0	1	2	3
Columns Totals				
Total Score (Sum of Column Totals)				

Which of the questions in the form describe experiences that have been present for you at times in your life when you have felt down or depressed, even if you use different words to describe what you were experiencing?

_____

_____

_____

_____

_____

_____

These questions are linked to the criteria that are used to diagnose what mental health professionals call major depression. These criteria are used to diagnose major depression at any time in a person's life, for women and for men.

Recognizing depression can be more challenging or confusing during pregnancy or postpartum. Some of the experiences are clearly different from typical prenatal and postpartum experiences (e.g., recurrent thoughts of death and suicide), whereas others often overlap with typical prenatal and postpartum experiences (e.g., fatigue or loss of energy).

To distinguish whether the experience of these symptoms is a warning sign that a woman is nearing or entering the territory of depression during pregnancy or when parenting a baby, mental health professionals pay attention to the specific symptoms, but also to these three dimensions:

- The number of symptoms

- The frequency and duration of the symptoms

- The degree to which the symptoms are associated with impairment

Thus, when mental health professionals define "an episode of major depression," they are referring to a time during which at least five of these symptoms (of which one must be the first or second) are present for most of the day, nearly every day, for at least 2 weeks. In addition, mental health professionals pay attention to the way in which these symptoms affect a person's ability to carry out her normal daily activities. For major depression during pregnancy or postpartum, a woman's ability to carry out normal daily activities is impaired, which may include caring for herself or her baby.

Even though a total of five symptoms and specific duration and impairment criteria are required to diagnose major depression, this doesn't mean that fewer symptoms or less frequent occurrence isn't important. In fact, there is good evidence that even a few symptoms that linger after a past episode of depression can be troubling for people.

In addition, it's common for problems of anxiety and worry to go along with depression during pregnancy and postpartum, as at other times. Most moms worry about their babies and their ability to care for their babies at some times, so mental health professionals focus on particular questions to help identify when worries have become more problematic than the kind of typical worries that many pregnant women and new moms experience. Mental health professionals pay attention to how many worries moms are experiencing and how difficult it is to control worrying. Mental health professionals also pay attention to times at which moms may experience a lot of intense physical sensations that come out of the blue and that cause a lot of worry or concern. Finally, some mothers experience recurrent thoughts or images, often about the baby, that are intrusive and disturbing and may experience compulsions to get rid of these thoughts with particular actions. In all of these cases, mental health professionals pay attention to how often these worries or anxieties occur and how much they are getting in the way of carrying out normal daily activities.

We will have an opportunity to explore in more detail the symptoms and experiences that are part of the territory of depression for you, specifically, in Class 6. For now, it's valuable to have a general understanding of the experience of depression during pregnancy and postpartum.

Daily Practice for Lesson 3

Talk with your support person about what you learned in this class.

◆ Discuss the territory of depression, anxiety, and your own "Top 10." You may share this with your support person in conversation, and you also might ask the person to read this part of the chapter and your notes. Record your reflections in your Practice Journal.

Choose a new daily routine activity to practice mindfulness in daily life.

◆ Continuing to bring mindfulness to your daily activities provides an important foundation on which we will build in later classes. You may select from the list on page 52 or follow the instructions for the "being with baby" practice (use the written instructions from Class 3 if you're pregnant or Track 11, "Being with Baby," if you're postpartum). Notice and record in your Practice Journal any thoughts or feelings that arise as you do the daily practice.

Daily Practice Summary

To recap, we invite you to do the following daily practices and record your experiences in your Practice Journal.

Lesson 1

• On days 1, 3, 5, and 7, do a sitting practice. Practice with 25 minutes of mindful breathing, using Track 8 for the "25-Minute Sitting Meditation" practice (or on very busy days, Track 7 for the "10-Minute Breathing Meditation" practice).

• On days 2, 4, and 6, do a movement practice. If you select the yoga practice, use the "25-Minute Yoga Practice" (Video 3) or on especially busy days the "10-Minute Yoga

Practice" (Video 2). If you select walking, listen and practice along with the 8-minute mindful "Walking Meditation" instructions (Track 9).

- Briefly record in your Practice Journal the sensations, thoughts, or emotions you notice and reflect on your experience with using the steps of the OPEN acronym.

Lesson 2

- Practice using the 3-minute breathing space three times a day, at set times that you've decided on in advance, and record the number of times you practice by circling "3MBS."

- Practice using the coping 3-minute breathing space during difficult situations. Record the number of times you practice by circling "Coping 3MBS" and note any comments/ difficulties.

- For the 3-minute breathing space, you may use the guided instructions (Track 10: "3-Minute Breathing Space") or the brief "reminder" instruction sheet from Class 3 (on page 77). For the coping 3-minute breathing space, review the instructions for the coping 3MBS on page 97.

Lesson 3

- Choose a new activity in your daily life. You may select from the list on page 52 or follow the instructions for the "being with baby" practice (use the written instructions from Class 3, on page 78, if you're pregnant or Track 11, "Being with Baby," if you're postpartum). Notice and record in your Practice Journal any thoughts or feelings that arise as you do the daily practice.

Circle of Support

- On at least 1 day, talk with your support person about what you learned from this chapter and what you're noticing in your daily practices, especially in relation to the territory of depression, anxiety, and your "Top 10." Record any reflections based on these conversations in the Circle of Support Reflections.

Practice Journal

	Day 1	Day 2	Day 3
Lesson 1 Practice Reflections: What did you notice in your sitting or movement practice today? Remember to alternate between these two from day to day. Did you use the steps of the OPEN acronym, and what did you notice if so?			
Example: *Today I decided to do the walking exercise. Most of the time, when I'm walking, I am mentally a million miles away, planning things or getting stuck in thinking about problems. Today, though, I noticed the feeling of my legs moving and the firmness of placing my feet on the sidewalk with each step. I didn't experience a lot of difficulty, so I didn't use the OPEN skills, but I did review them so that they are familiar and accessible. . . . I know difficulty and uncertainty is bound to pop up before too long!*			
Lesson 2 Practice Reflections: Three-minute breathing space (3MBS). Circle each time you do one of your three daily 3MBS practices and when you use the Coping 3MBS. Note any comments/difficulties.			
	3MBS 3MBS 3MBS Coping 3MBS	3MBS 3MBS 3MBS Coping 3MBS	3MBS 3MBS 3MBS Coping 3MBS
Lesson 3 Practice Reflections: Record here any thoughts or feelings you notice in your mindfulness of daily activity or your "being with baby" practice.			
Example: *I've had a hard time with the "being with baby" practice. Most of the time it's hard to tell whether the baby is moving or I have gas or something! Today, however, I felt the baby kick! It was definitely a kick or a punch. It was sudden and pretty noticeable. I felt relief and excitement.*			

110

Practice Journal

Day 4	Day 5	Day 6	Day 7
3MBS	3MBS	3MBS	3MBS
3MBS	3MBS	3MBS	3MBS
3MBS	3MBS	3MBS	3MBS
Coping 3MBS	Coping 3MBS	Coping 3MBS	Coping 3MBS

Circle of Support Reflections

What did you notice in connecting with your support person this week?

CLASS 5

Thoughts Are Not Facts

It isn't what we say or think that defines us, but what we do.
—Jane Austen

This chapter includes the following three lessons:

1. **Our minds often "add on" to experience with thoughts that can make tough times even tougher.** We invite you to begin to notice how your mind adds on to experience and to explore the possibility that "thoughts are not facts."

2. **How we feel, physically and emotionally, can have a powerful influence on the point of view we take about a situation**. We help you begin to explore the connections among moods, thoughts, and points of view.

3. **All of the skills of mindfulness that you have developed provide a strong foundation for working with particularly difficult negative thoughts**. We invite you to practice the 3-minute breathing space, followed by two approaches that many have found helpful in working with particularly difficult, negative "add-on" thoughts.

Lesson 1. Adding On

Often when we face difficulty or uncertainty, we add on thoughts. You may be wondering, what's an "add-on" thought? See if you recognize any of these:

- In the middle of the afternoon at work, Aleeta realized, "I'm thoroughly exhausted and don't know how I'm going to get through the rest of the day," and then added on "I'm never going to get any sleep and the baby hasn't even arrived!"

- In the restaurant bathroom, trying to change her son's diaper, Mina observed, "It's really hard to change his diaper, and he tries to squirm away from me; I have very little control!," and then added on "I can just see the other women walking in here and judging, thinking what a terrible mother I am."

Similar to these mothers, you may add on thoughts about the future:

- This is going to last forever.
- This is never going to change.
- Things will always be this way.

You also may add on thoughts about yourself:

- I'm not good enough.
- I'm a failure.
- I'm a bad mother.

When you turn to your mindfulness practice, you might even add on such thoughts about that experience:

- I shouldn't be thinking that.
- I'm not doing this right.
- This isn't working.

In each of these cases, you may be adding on to the specific experience by drawing general conclusions about the situation, the future, or yourself *and* stating these conclusions as facts. You may relate to these thoughts as though they are *the truth*.

If you have experienced depression or anxiety, your thoughts can become like a campaign directed against yourself and your future. Negative, self-critical thoughts are like constant ads flashing on the background of the mind's screen: "I'm a failure." "My life is a mess." "It's just not worth it." "I'm unattractive." "I'll never know what to do as a new mom."

At times, "add-on" thoughts even pop up when we're having pleasurable experiences, including thoughts like "I don't deserve this" or "I'm being selfish." Pleasurable experiences can slip, without your awareness, into stressful ones as your mind adds on thoughts about how infrequently you experience pleasure or how fleeting the experience can be.

These kinds of "add-on" thoughts can be particularly powerful, with a force capable of carrying you far from the present moment.

They can pull you into a downward spiral that can leave you feeling much worse very quickly. The spiral starts with thoughts that are anchored in our direct experiences—sensations, emotions, and experiences in the present moment—and then the "add-on" thoughts, often very self-critical, carry us into the past or the future and downward into feeling down, depleted, or overwhelmed.

During pregnancy and parenting, there are so many times you may be particularly vulnerable to this "add-on" thinking: when you haven't slept, when your home demands and work demands are in conflict, when someone criticizes your ideas or actions as a mom, when you come up against physical challenges like weight gain or mobility restrictions, when your partner is not understanding or attentive to how best to support you. During these times you may add on thoughts—and often ones that don't serve you well.

Elaine found herself caught in a downward spiral one afternoon. She observed: "I'm so tired. The baby is really hard to settle today. He won't let me put him down for a moment without fussing." All of these thoughts were closely anchored in her experience and observations in the present moment . . . and then came the "add-on" thoughts!

In rapid succession, her mind generated the following, which pulled her down into feeling even more exhausted and overwhelmed:

- This keeps happening; it's every day.

- This is as bad as the feeding problems when he was born.

- I can't get through another day of this.

- The stuff I read online says he should be napping more.

- I don't know what I'm doing.

 In your practice today, we invite you to look for the ways in which you add on thoughts. As you identify your "add-on" thoughts, you may discover opportunities to learn that you don't have to believe all the thoughts your mind comes up with.

Practice Now

Let's practice now. We invite you to bring to mind a difficult or troubling thought or situation—some situation that carries intense emotion, such as sadness, fear, shame, or anger. As you practice, notice any "add-on" thoughts that arrive. They might be about the situation you bring to mind (e.g., "This is never going to change"), or they might be simply about the experience of doing the mindfulness practice (e.g., "My back is killing me; I can't sit here for one more second"). Take a few moments to prepare your space, and when you're ready, please use audio Track 12, "Difficult Emotions," for a 10-minute guided practice. When you're finished, please return to reflect on your experience.

Reflections on Practice

What sensations, emotions, or thoughts were present as you brought the difficulty to mind?

_____

_____

_____

_____

"I felt strong waves of nausea."

"I felt so frustrated."

"I had the thought that I forgot to call the doctor."

In what ways did your mind add on to your experience with conclusions, predictions, and other statements of "fact"? Did you add on thoughts of pushing away or dwelling on particular experiences?

_____

_____

_____

_____

Circle of Mothers

"I definitely added on thoughts about the future, like 'I will never be able to handle things at work tomorrow if I still feel like this.'"

"I added on thoughts for sure—'I can't stand this; nothing can help us.'"

As you reflect on your vision for staying well during pregnancy, postpartum, and beyond, how might awareness of the ways in which your mind adds on thoughts support you along the staying-well path?

_____

_____

_____

_____

_____

_____

Circle of Mothers

"It seems like bringing this awareness to what you're thinking and how you're adding on thoughts opens up a lot of possibilities, like maybe it's not written in stone that I can't function at work when I'm tired. That's an extra thought my mind is adding on."

"The whole thoughts-are-not-facts thing has helped me a lot in dealing with the worry about my son's illness. It's helped me not be so freaked out when things come up at the doctor's office. Without that, it's like the thoughts run the show 24/7. Now I know how to get a little more grounded in how I feel physically and tell myself that I'm feeling afraid but the awful scenarios about what my thoughts are saying will happen are not necessarily true."

Bring Attention to Sensations in Your Body

When the mind is very busy adding on and telling stories about a situation, a core skill is shifting the focus of your attention back into the present moment by grounding your attention in sensations that you feel in your body. Focusing on how you feel, moment to moment, in the body can provide another place to stand when the mind is very busy adding on thoughts. Your mind may be very loud and compelling, with many "add-on" thoughts about, for example, how you will never sleep through the night. Bringing your attention to the direct, immediate sensations in the body—heaviness in the shoulders, tightness around the eyes, and so forth—can provide a place for the mind to settle. Other "add-on" thoughts may be loud and compelling about some of your worst fears, such as your baby's health or conflict with your partner and fears of being alone. Bringing your attention to sensations like tightness in the chest, agitation in your arms or legs, and gripping in your belly also can provide a place for the mind to settle.

Notice Change, Including the Seemingly Irrelevant

Many of the mind's "add-on" thoughts suggest that things always have been or always will be the same. By bringing our attention back to the present moment in the body, we may discover that our experience is always changing, even if only subtly. Thus, although the tightness around the eyes may not "go away" as you notice it and the pit in your stomach might not immediately release, the intensity may shift from moment to moment, reminding you that things are rarely absolute and permanent. In these ways, grounding your attention in the body can be a helpful response when the mind is busy adding on. It's helpful to connect to the immediate experience that things change, even if it's changing sensation that seems irrelevant—such as minor fluctuations in tightness in the brow or belly. Noticing these small changes in your body helps you "know" something very important: thoughts like "This will never change" are not absolute truth. If you practice that with thoughts about sensations like tightness in the eyes (e.g., "I'm going to have this headache forever!"), you will be more skilled when faced with thoughts about more weighty matters (e.g., "I'm always going to feel alone in this marriage").

Greet Thoughts as Visitors

The essential skill to develop is to go from automatically accepting the "add-on" thoughts as truth to seeing them as events in the mind. Using metaphors, like thoughts as visitors, can be a helpful way to respond to the mind's habit of adding on. As moms or moms-to-be, you've probably experienced friends or relatives wanting to come to visit. Some of these visitors are welcome, and we greet them eagerly. In contrast, other visitors are less appealing and impose themselves on us. We may tolerate them, feeling a sense of heaviness when they arrive and a sense of relief when they go. In each case, though, they are just visiting. We're not inviting them to move in or pushing them away when they knock at the door. We can practice this with our thoughts. Just because they show up at the front door does not mean that you have to prepare the guest room, nor does it mean that you have to secure all the locks. We can't stop our thoughts from visiting, but we can acknowledge their presence and then let them go. You may find it helpful to keep in mind this metaphor. Many people also appreciate the poem "The Guest House" for the images it provides and the invitation to experience this welcoming stance.

The Guest House

This being human is a guest house.
Every morning a new arrival.
A joy, a depression, a meanness,
some momentary awareness comes
as an unexpected visitor.
Welcome and entertain them all!
Even if they are a crowd of sorrows,
who violently sweep your house
empty of its furniture,
still, treat each guest honorably.
He may be clearing you out
for some new delight.
The dark thought, the shame, the malice.
meet them at the door laughing and invite them in.
Be grateful for whatever comes.
because each has been sent
as a guide from beyond.
    —Rumi (Coleman Barks, translator)

Remind Yourself, Thoughts Are Not Facts

Just because thoughts arise does not make them facts, even though, in the moment, the way you are feeling can make the thought powerfully convincing! Many mothers have told us that the simple phrase "thoughts are not facts" has been a powerful support to them in responding wisely to challenging thoughts and caring for themselves.

Daily Practice for Lesson 1

Do a 10-minute, guided "Mindfully Responding to Difficulty" practice each day, using audio Track 12, "Difficult Emotions."

◆ Bring to mind a difficult or troubling thought or situation—some situation that carries for you intense emotion, such as sadness, fear, shame, or anger. Notice, in particular, any "add-on" thinking that arises and how you respond to such thinking—do you identify the process of "add-on" thinking, or do you respond to specific thoughts as facts? Briefly record in your Practice Journal the sensations, thoughts, or emotions—and any "add-on" thinking!—that you notice each time you practice.

◆ Remember to be patient with yourself as you do these practices. The habits of adding on may have been with you for many, many years. It takes practice and time to notice the "add-on" thoughts as they're occurring. Even noticing a few occasions over the course of the next week is a great step to working differently with such patterns.

Lesson 2. Points of View

It's possible to see a situation from many points of view. Many different factors shape your point of view. During pregnancy and postpartum, your point of view can be powerfully shaped by your emotional state at the time, and in turn, your point of view is a powerful source of "add-on" thoughts. Let's explore this together now.

Practice Now

Take a moment to read over the following description and then close your eyes and imagine yourself in that situation as vividly as possible:

You are feeling down because you've just had an argument with a coworker. Shortly afterward, you see another coworker in the main office, and she rushes off quickly, saying she can't stop. What do you think?

Write down the thoughts that went through your mind.

_____

_____

_____

_____

_____

Now take a moment to read over the following description and then close your eyes and imagine yourself in that situation as vividly as possible:

You are feeling happy because you and a coworker have just been praised for good work. Shortly afterward, you see another coworker in the main office, and she rushes off quickly, saying she can't stop. What do you think?

Write down the thoughts that went through your mind.

_____

_____

_____

_____

_____

Let's continue this practice with another situation. Take a moment to read over the following description and then close your eyes and imagine yourself in that situation as vividly as possible:

You are feeling down because you have just had an argument with your spouse/partner. Shortly afterward, your baby wakes up from a nap, crying intensely. You are trying to soothe your baby, who keeps crying and doesn't settle down. What do you think?

Write down the thoughts that went through your mind.

_____

_____

_____

_____

_____

Last scenario: take a moment to read over the following description and then close your eyes and imagine yourself in that situation as vividly as possible:

You are feeling happy because you and your spouse/partner have just shared a nice dinner. Shortly afterward, your baby wakes up from a nap, crying intensely. You are trying to soothe your baby, who keeps crying and doesn't settle down. What do you think?

Write down the thoughts that went through your mind.

_____

_____

_____

_____

_____

Please consider the thoughts you listed in response to the two situations, one related to a work setting and the other to home. What strikes you as you read over your responses? How similar are your responses to these situations to what happens in your everyday life?

_____

_____

_____

_____

_____

_____

Circle
of Mothers

Read the responses of the circle of mothers to the same scenarios.

"If that first scenario happened to me when I was feeling down, I would walk away, and I would spin that tape until I saw them again, and I would say things like 'He must be really upset with me.' Even in the second situation with the baby crying, some kind of really personal negative tape would start playing if I were coming to the situation with the point of view of feeling down. I never know how to stop that tape once it gets started. I never considered that it was influenced by my mood, like just if you were in a positive versus a negative mood before the situation even happened. Definitely, if I'm feeling good, the tape doesn't really get started."

"A lot of things—like did I eat or sleep enough that day—have a big impact on how I react. If I'm feeling down because I was up a lot with the baby and I haven't had time to even take a shower in days, and then if my husband comes home and goes right to the kitchen to get something to eat, I can get really irritated, like why doesn't he care about the baby or me. But if I am coming with a more positive point of view because I'm feeling happy about the baby being really sweet and taking a long nap and I was able to take care of things, and even take a shower, then even if he does the same thing when he gets home, I'm okay with it. I don't take it personally."

Emotions Love Themselves

Our friend and colleague Marsha Linehan often says, "Emotions love themselves." What she means by this is that a particular emotion will tend to trigger thoughts that keep that emotion present. So, when you're sad, your mind is likely to generate sad thoughts and the feelings of sadness are more likely to persist in the form of a depressed mood. When you're worried, your mind generates worry thoughts that are likely to sustain the worry. Thus, how you are feeling sets the stage for particular thoughts. This can be especially powerful when faced with ambiguous or uncertain situations. At such times the mind tends to "fill in the blanks" in ways that are consistent with the emotion you're experiencing. Thus, if you're feeling overwhelmed and alone in caring for a fussy baby, and your partner comes home late from work, your mind may be more likely to generate "add-on" thoughts like "My partner doesn't care about how I'm feeling or what I need." You fill in the blanks with emotion-consistent thoughts. In contrast, if you're feeling happy, you may be more likely to generate "add-on" thoughts like "My partner must be exhausted after such a long day" or perhaps more likely to refrain from drawing conclusions at all and simply gather the missing information with questions like "How was your day? What kept you so late?"

Don't Believe Everything You Think

When your mind is generating a lot of "emotion-consistent" thoughts, it can be harder to see each thought as a thought. They just feel "true." Also, your physical state can influence the extent to which you believe your thoughts. If you're physically exhausted by the experience of pregnancy or caring for a newborn, thoughts can be a lot more convincing than at other times. It's very hard at such times to "step back" to see thoughts for what they are: events in the mind. As Sade explained: "I remind myself that thoughts are not facts every day. That is just one of the most important things I learned. So, when I start to get lost in my thoughts and think, 'This is going to happen, and if this happens, this is going to happen, and then it's going to be horrible,' I step back and see the spiral of thoughts for what they are. When I see that I'm carried away, I step back and check in with myself about how I'm feeling physically and what emotions I'm feeling. I focus on any signs of my mood or exhaustion or hunger, all of those things that make me start to believe everything I'm thinking. And I remind myself that thoughts are not facts. It gives me the confidence that I can take control of my life instead of getting carried away by the thoughts."

Daily Practice for Lesson 2

This week we invite you to build on the practices we introduced in the last sessions of mindfulness in daily life. Bringing mindfulness to your daily activities provides an important foundation for developing an action plan for wellness that we'll build on in later classes.

◆ Choose a new activity in your daily life. You may select something from the list on page 52, follow the instructions for the "being with baby" practice when you feel the movements of the baby or physical sensations of being pregnant (page 78), or, if you have a new baby, you can use Track 11, "Being with Baby."

◆ During your practice, we invite you to pay close attention to any situations in which you experience strong emotions. Ask yourself if you're coming to the situation with a particular point of view that is, itself, influenced by your mood or your body state. How have you been feeling emotionally and physically? Have you felt scared, happy, angry, and/or stressed? Are you tired or hungry? How are these mood and physical states shaping your point of view? Notice and record any reflections in your Practice Journal.

Lesson 3. The 3-Minute Breathing Space and "Add-On" Thinking

When emotions are intense or you are physically drained, which often is true during pregnancy and parenting, it can be helpful to have additional tools to respond to difficult points of view and particularly negative or powerful "add-on" thoughts.

In this lesson, we invite you to practice with two approaches that many have found helpful in working with particularly difficult, negative "add-on" thoughts. Both of these approaches begin with the 3-minute breathing space to invite a balanced, open state of mind. Following this, the first approach relies on writing down thoughts and the second approach relies on asking questions.

Practice Now

Let's practice now. Bring something to mind that is difficult—although not the most difficult thing you can imagine. Perhaps consider a situation that is about a 5 on a difficulty scale of 0 (not difficult at all) to 10 (the most difficult ever).

Take a 3-minute breathing space, supported by listening to Track 10, "3-Minute Breathing Space," or reviewing the written instructions on page 77, as you bring to mind this level-5 difficulty. When you're finished, return to practice with these next two approaches for working with particularly difficult, negative "add-on" thoughts.

1. *Writing down the add-on thoughts:* Often, writing down the thoughts lets you see them in a way that is less emotional and overwhelming. Also, the pause between having the thought and writing it down can give you a moment to reflect on the process of adding on or filling in the blanks and the power of such thoughts. Writing them down can help you remember: thoughts are not facts! What "add-on" thoughts did you notice as you brought to mind the level-5 difficulty?

_____

_____

_____

_____

_____

2. *Asking questions:* Holding the negative, "add-on" thoughts in awareness, with an attitude of gentle interest, ask yourself as many of the following questions as are helpful in eliciting a sense of curiosity. You also may experiment with going back to the breath after bringing each question to mind. Ask yourself, Am I . . .

  - confusing a thought with a fact?
  - jumping to conclusions?
  - thinking in black-and-white terms?
  - overestimating disaster?
  - mind reading/crystal-ball gazing?
  - judging myself?
  - setting unrealistically high standards for myself?
  - expecting perfection?
  - condemning myself totally because of one thing?
  - concentrating on my weaknesses and forgetting my strengths?
  - blaming myself for something that isn't my fault?

The key is to practice bringing an attitude of gentle interest and curiosity—even with very difficult, negative thoughts. Circle the questions that were most helpful to you in encouraging curiosity rather than simply accepting thoughts as facts.

Reflections on Practice

What did you notice in writing down your "add-on" thoughts or working with the list of questions?

_____

_____

_____

_____

_____

_____

Circle of Mothers

Taking the 3-minute breathing space is a lifesaver. And then writing down the thoughts that were still there after the third step. . . . it was good, literally, to get those thoughts out of my head and onto paper!"

"Writing down my thoughts gave me a moment to pause, and then, when I started to use the questions, I almost had to laugh. I was saying 'yes' to almost all of them!"

"When I stood back and read what I had written, I could see that all of my thoughts were the same add-on . . . basically criticizing myself for not doing things well, expecting perfection, all of that."

As you reflect on your vision for staying well during pregnancy, postpartum, and beyond, how might these ways of responding to "add-on" thoughts support you along the staying-well path?

_____

_____

_____

_____

_____

_____

Circle of Mothers

"I have used this practice a bunch of times. In fact, I started keeping an 'add-on' journal so that I could look back on what I wrote. I just put the date and whatever thoughts were there when I had a chance to write them down. I started to notice that it was the same thoughts popping up over and over in different situations. So now I'm more able to recognize, 'There's that old thought again.' It just doesn't carry the same weight."

"The 'add-on' thoughts are like a slippery slope for me. It's literally like sliding down a hill of ice. It used to be like I wouldn't even realize I had started to slide until I was well down the hill. Using the 3-minute breathing space helps me catch my breath, and then using those questions is a great tool. It's like an ice pick that I can use to stop my fall. Now, when I'm sliding, I ask myself, 'Am I confusing a thought with a fact (again!)? Am I jumping to conclusions?' With each question, it's like I'm digging that ice pick into the side of the slippery slope and stopping the slide down. I definitely still slip, but I'm catching myself earlier and earlier as I practice this more and more."

"I love the 3-minute breathing space. It is so short, and I can use it in so many situations. Expanding the practice to notice 'add-on' thoughts helps me so much. When I feel like I'm beginning to drown in this big whirlpool of thoughts and emotions, taking a 3-minute breathing space and then writing down the 'add-on' thoughts helped me see that I was either in shallow water and could stand or that I had a life preserver and was in no real danger."

Daily Practice for Lesson 3

◆ Practice using the 3-minute breathing space three times a day, at set times that you have decided on in advance, and record the number of times you practice by circling "3MBS."

◆ Practice using the coping 3-minute breathing space during difficult situations. Record the number of times you practice by circling "Coping 3MBS." You may use the guided instructions (Track 10, "3-Minute Breathing Space"), or you can use the brief "reminder" instructions from Class 4 (page 97). When difficult thoughts are present, experiment with using the approaches of writing down thoughts or asking questions.

Daily Practice Summary

To recap, we invite you to do the following daily practices and record your experiences in your Practice Journal.

Lesson 1

- Do a "Mindfully Responding to Difficulty" practice each day, using audio Track 12, "Difficult Emotions," which is an approximately 10-minute guided practice. Notice, in particular, any "add-on" thinking that arises and how you respond to such thinking—do you identify the process of "add-on" thinking or do you respond to specific thoughts as facts?

- Briefly record the sensations, thoughts, or emotions—and any "add-on" thinking—that you notice each time you practice in your Practice Journal.

Lesson 2

- Choose a new activity in your daily life. You may either select from the list on page 52 or follow the instructions for the "being with baby" practice when you feel the movements of the baby or physical sensations of being pregnant.

- During your practice, we invite you to notice, in particular, connections between your point of view and any "add-on" thoughts, as well as the ways in which such thoughts might be influenced by how you feel, emotionally or physically (e.g., feeling sad or scared or happy or tired or hungry).

- Notice and record in your Practice Journal any thoughts or feelings that arise as you do the daily practice.

Lesson 3

- Practice using the 3-minute breathing space three times a day, at set times that you've decided on in advance, and record the number of times you practice by circling "3MBS."

- Practice using the coping 3-minute breathing space during difficult situations. Record the number of times you practice by circling "Coping 3MBS" and note any comments or difficulties. When difficult thoughts are present, you may experiment with using the approaches of writing down thoughts and asking questions. To begin, simply write down the thoughts that are present in your mind. This can help you step back and get a little more space from the thoughts. Sometimes, the process of writing down thoughts can help you remember that thoughts are not facts.

_____

_____

_____

_____

_____

- Once you've written down the thoughts, invite an attitude of gentle interest and curiosity by asking yourself some questions. Ask yourself as many of the following questions as are helpful in inviting a sense of curiosity and openness. You also may experiment with bringing your awareness to your breathing, even just one inhale and one exhale, after asking each question. If you find that some questions are more helpful to you than others, we encourage you to highlight or circle those so that they are even more accessible to you when difficult thoughts come up in the future.

  Am I . . .

  - confusing a thought with a fact?
  - jumping to conclusions?
  - thinking in black-and-white terms?
  - overestimating disaster?
  - mind reading/crystal-ball gazing?
  - judging myself?
  - setting unrealistically high standards for myself?
  - expecting perfection?
  - condemning myself totally because of one thing?
  - concentrating on my weaknesses and forgetting my strengths?
  - blaming myself for something that isn't my fault?

Circle of Support

- On at least one day, talk with your support person about what you learned from this chapter and what you are noticing in your daily practices. Record any reflections based on these conversations in the Circle of Support Reflections.

Practice Journal

	Day 1	Day 2	Day 3
Lesson 1 Practice Reflections: What did you notice in your practice of mindfully responding to difficulty today? Remember to record any "add-on" thoughts that you noticed.			
Example: *I spent the whole day on the couch. I was exhausted! I noticed a lot of add-on thoughts: I should be exercising, I am going to gain so much weight, the house is a mess and I should be on top of it. So many shoulds!! I noticed them and pretty much let them go. I ended up sleeping most of the day.*			
Lesson 2 Practice Reflections: Briefly note any reflections during your mindfulness of daily activity or your "being with baby" practice. Reflect on any occasions when your emotional or physical state shaped your point of view.			
Example: *I was so happy about finally getting the things for the baby's room. I felt a lot of sensation in my belly, which might have been aggravating if I were in a different point of view. Today, though, I was feeling so happy. I closed my eyes to feel baby, and I began talking to him, telling him that he would soon be here and this room was all set up with a lot of love. I could feel him moving around as I spoke. It was beautiful and peaceful.*			
Lesson 3 Practice Reflections: Do the 3-minute breathing space (3MBS). Please circle each time you do one of your three daily 3MBS practices and when you use the coping 3MBS. Use the writing down of "add-on' thoughts or asking questions as needed.			
Example: (3MBS) (3MBS) (3MBS) (Coping 3MBS) *Add-on thoughts: Will this ever get easier? This is going to push me over the edge.* *Questions: Am I jumping to conclusions? Yes!*	3MBS 3MBS 3MBS Coping 3MBS	3MBS 3MBS 3MBS Coping 3MBS	3MBS 3MBS 3MBS Coping 3MBS

Practice Journal

Day 4	Day 5	Day 6	Day 7
3MBS	3MBS	3MBS	3MBS
3MBS	3MBS	3MBS	3MBS
3MBS	3MBS	3MBS	3MBS
Coping 3MBS	Coping 3MBS	Coping 3MBS	Coping 3MBS

Circle of Support Reflections

What did you notice in connecting with your support person this week?

CLASS 6

How Can I Best Take Care of Myself?

Radical self-care is quantum, and it radiates out from you into the atmosphere like a little fresh air. It's a huge gift to the world.

—Anne Lamott

This chapter includes the following three lessons:

1. **The practice of lovingkindness can help you bring gentleness and self-care into your life, even during tough times**. We invite you to begin to learn this practice—building the skill of being kind with yourself.

2. **Bringing mindful awareness to daily routines allows you to learn a lot about the connections between what you do and how you feel**. We invite you to discover some of these connections and explore how you might use this knowledge to care for yourself.

3. **Everyone has warning signs that signal when depression, anxiety, and stress are beginning to take hold**. We guide you in recognizing your individual warning signs and using this information to care for yourself to stay well, including writing a letter to yourself in the future.

Lesson 1. Lovingkindness

Women often hold themselves to very high standards and judge themselves harshly for not meeting them. During the mindfulness practices that you have learned in our first five classes, you've had opportunities to practice the important skill of being gentle and caring instead of critical toward yourself whenever your attention was caught by difficult thoughts, emotions, or sensations. In many small moments, you've practiced gently returning your attention to the breath without judging yourself for the wandering of your mind.

Today the practice of being kind and gentle with yourself becomes the primary focus of meditation. In this first lesson we invite you to learn a practice called "lovingkindness meditation." You can strengthen the skill of lovingkindness with both sitting and walking practices. In each case we will work with a set of phrases that you will be asked to repeat silently in your mind. There are three sets of phrases, each of which aims to direct your mind and heart to the possibility of wellness for yourself, your baby, and other loved ones in your life.

- "May I be filled with lovingkindness. May I treat myself with kindness in good times and in hard times. May I be well and live with ease."

- "May my baby be surrounded with lovingkindness. May I respond to my baby with kindness in good times and in hard times. May my baby be well and live with ease."

- "May you be surrounded with lovingkindness. May you treat yourself with kindness in good times and in hard times. May you be well and live with ease."

Practice Now

Take a few moments to prepare your space. When you're ready, listen to the "Lovingkindness Meditation Introduction" (Track 14) and then use the audio recording for the "20-Minute Lovingkindness Meditation Sitting Practice" (Track 15) to guide your practice. When you've completed the sitting lovingkindness practice, please continue with Track 16 for the "10-Minute Lovingkindness Walking Practice." When you're finished with both, please return to reflect on your experience.

Reflections on Practice

What did you notice while doing the lovingkindness practices?

_____

_____

_____

_____

Circle of Mothers

"I felt a lot of love as soon as I started, and I thought about my grandmother. It really was like a sense of love or peace filling my heart."

"I had a hard time focusing. Repeating each of the phrases felt forced when directed toward myself. I tried to bring in the idea that this was a gift to myself and allow myself to embrace that gift, but I didn't feel much of anything when I was focusing on myself. When I shifted to my baby, my partner, and the world, everything changed. I felt waves of peace and calm."

"I felt awkward, maybe a little guilty, like I should be doing something else, but then I thought it was worth just following along with the instructions."

In what ways does this practice differ from your typical experience of relating to yourself?

_____

_____

_____

_____

Circle of Mothers

"Typically, I'm hard on myself. My 'add-on' thoughts are usually things like 'You can't do anything right,' and I don't even realize I'm saying that to myself a lot of the time. Learning the lovingkindness instructions is really different. It feels calming to me. I don't think I've ever said things to myself like 'May I treat myself with kindness in good times and in hard times. May I be well and live with ease.' It's about as close to a 180 turn as I can imagine from what's been typical."

"I'm my own harshest and strictest critic. So, this didn't really change with my practice today. I have difficulty when the practice focuses on me. When it switches to my baby, I can more easily feel and emanate lovingkindness. The first part is just really hard for me; the habit of harsh self-criticism is pretty strong! I think it might take practice."

As you reflect on your vision for staying well during pregnancy, postpartum, and beyond, how might this practice support you along the staying-well path?

_____

_____

_____

_____

Circle of Mothers

"Treating myself with such harsh criticism is exhausting. It's become so normal that I don't really realize how exhausting it is anymore, but this practice helps me see how exhausting it is. I can imagine, over time, that doing this practice can help me begin to show lovingkindness toward myself. This is important for me so that I'm not so exhausted and run down. It's also important because I don't want to set an example for my child of being so mean to myself. I just hate to think of my daughter being so hard on herself one day."

"I use the lovingkindness meditation all the time from the class. I've always had a hard time asking people for help, and this meditation reminds me that it's okay to call for help. Often, if I think someone doesn't understand what I'm feeling, I tend to just pull away, isolate myself. With this practice, though, if I think about being kind to myself, it helps me pause for a moment and then actually reach out instead of pulling away."

"For me, the walking lovingkindness is a lifesaver. It's just so quick, and I can do it all the time when I'm walking the baby. I sync it up with my steps: 'May I be well. May you be well.' The other day, someone bumped the stroller while we were walking. Before this class, I would have gotten irritated, but it was kind of amazing, I just said quietly, 'May you be well' once he had passed by."

"I think repeating things like 'May I be well' reminds me to do things for myself, little things like pausing to rest for a few minutes instead of automatically going for another cup of coffee when I have so much to do. Or at the end of my pregnancy, I paid for the parking that was closer to my office because it made my mornings a lot easier."

Whatever You Feel Is Okay

All of the experiences women have while learning this practice are just fine. There is no one "right" way to feel while doing the lovingkindness practice. You don't have to force any part, and it's not a contest to see who can feel the most loving or calm. The only thing that matters is listening to the instructions and gently repeating the phrases, returning to them again and again when your attention wanders.

Giving and Receiving

Developing the skill of lovingkindness can help you bring balance between caring for others and caring for yourself. Many understand the value of self-care and yet find it a challenge to put such understanding into practice. The practice of lovingkindness reminds you of the balance between self and other. Anita voiced the experience of many women when she commented, "I really struggle with directing lovingkindness toward myself. I find it easier to do toward others. I think that the lovingkindness meditation exercise will eventually help me bring lovingkindness to myself." With repeated practice, directing lovingkindness toward yourself encourages you to not only give care but also open yourself to receiving it, including from yourself.

Connecting with Your Baby

One of the benefits of this practice during pregnancy and early parenting is the opportunity to pause and focus your attention on your connection with your baby. For some, this connection comes automatically, and for others the experience of pregnancy and adjusting to life as a new mom feels foreign and unfamiliar. The latter was true for Sophie. The sense of strangeness started to shift with doing the lovingkindness practice. She explained: "I have felt more closely and positively connected to my pregnancy with this practice than before. I have struggled with so many parts of being pregnant—gaining weight, feeling exhausted and sick, other people's expectations of how I should be feeling, and most of all this strange feeling that being pregnant is like having an alien growing inside me! The lovingkindness practice really helped me feel more positive about being pregnant and connect to this creature who is my baby. It's been a whole new experience."

Kindness Where Once Was Criticism

One mom who worked with us told us about a quote displayed in a friend's bathroom. It said, "It's hard to be happy when someone is mean to you all the time." Initially, she thought its message was to encourage people to be kind to others, and then she realized that the message might be even more powerful when applied to herself. It's hard to be happy when you're mean to yourself all the time. When facing common challenges of pregnancy or the postpartum—exhaustion, caring for a fussy baby, feeling overwhelmed—it is so easy to focus on what seems wrong about yourself instead of what seems right. An example of a common tendency would be facing a crying baby, which is tough enough, and then adding on beliefs like "What am I doing wrong?" or "I can't handle this." It's very easy to think that you are a bad mother or a bad person. At these times it can be especially helpful to turn to the practice of lovingkindness. This practice can invite tenderness and care into your daily life where there may have been judgment and criticism. Remember: "It's hard to be happy when someone (including you!) is mean to you all the time." The practice of lovingkindness can be a great support in coping with the tough times that moms often face and bringing a little more gentleness to the experience.

Daily Practice for Lesson 1

Practice the lovingkindness meditation each day, using the audio guides to support your practice.

◆ You have the option of doing either of the lovingkindness practices— sitting (Track 15) or walking (Track 16). You can alternate between them, do both each day, or choose one for the week. If it's helpful, you also can listen to the "Introduction to Lovingkindness Meditation" again to remind you of the intention of these practices (Track 14). Briefly record what you notice during your practice in your Practice Journal.

Lesson 2. What Do You Do Each Day?

Paying attention to what you do each day builds on all of the mindfulness practices you've learned and is a critical part of staying well. Seeing the connections between what you do and how you feel gives you access to valuable knowledge that you can use to help you stay well.

Let's begin with writing down the activities you do on a typical day. Bring to mind a recent day to help you recall the specific details of what you were doing, with whom, where, and any other pertinent details.

Here's an example of the morning activities of Ellen, the mother of a 5-year-old son and a 2-month-old daughter:

	Activity	Nourishing	Depleting
5:00 A.M.	Waking up, thinking about my day		
6:00 A.M.	Getting up, making coffee, packing lunches, hearing the baby cry, changing diaper		
7:00 A.M.	Waking up my son and getting him and the baby dressed and out the door		
8:00 A.M.	Driving to school		

Notice that Ellen wrote specific activities for each hour rather than simply recording "taking care of the kids" between 6:00 and 9:00 A.M. It's helpful to write down enough detail that you have a clear sense of what you were doing but not so much detail that the recording itself is a burden.

For now, turn to the next page and just focus on the "Activity" column and write down your daily activities. We will guide you in completing the other columns in a few moments. Also, if your weekday and weekends are very different, you also might make a copy of the form on page 140 (information on printing extra forms can be found at the end of the Contents) so that you can write down the activities of a typical weekday and weekend day.

Now that you've completed the activity column, we want to explain how to complete the "Nourishing" and "Depleting" columns. There are two sets of questions to keep in mind:

1. **Does this activity *nourish* me?** Does doing this activity give me energy, peace of mind, or help me feel replenished? If the answer is "yes," you may put a check mark in the Nourishing column.
2. **Does this activity *deplete* me?** Does doing this activity drain my energy, stress me out, or bring me down? If the answer is "yes," you may put a check mark in the Depleting column.

It's okay if you place checks in both the "Nourishing" and "Depleting" columns for the same activity. Some activities are both.

The example below shows what Ellen recorded: some hours contained activities that were clearly depleting or clearly nourishing, whereas the 7:00–8:00 a.m. hour had elements of both.

	Activity	Nourishing	Depleting
5:00 A.M.	Waking up, thinking about my day		✓
6:00 A.M.	Getting up, making coffee, packing lunches, hearing the baby cry, changing diaper		✓
7:00 A.M.	Waking up my son and getting him and the baby dressed and out the door	✓	✓
8:00 A.M.	Driving to school	✓	✓

Now return to page 140 and place checks for "Nourishing," "Depleting," or both, for each activity listed.

Looking over your list on page 140, what did you notice? Anything surprising? What about the balance of nourishing and depleting activities?

_____

_____

_____

Noticing Daily Activities

	Activity	Nourishing	Depleting
5:00 A.M.			
6:00 A.M.			
7:00 A.M.			
8:00 A.M.			
9:00 A.M.			
10:00 A.M.			
11:00 A.M.			
12:00 P.M.			
1:00 P.M.			
2:00 P.M.			
3:00 P.M.			
4:00 P.M.			
5:00 P.M.			
6:00 P.M.			
7:00 P.M.			
8:00 P.M.			
9:00 P.M.			
10:00 P.M.			
11:00 P.M.			
12:00 A.M.			
1:00 A.M–4:00 A.M.			

From *Expecting Mindfully: Nourish Your Emotional Well-Being and Prevent Depression during Pregnancy and Postpartum,* by Sona Dimidjian and Sherryl H. Goodman. Copyright © 2019 The Guilford Press. Purchasers of this book can photocopy and/or download additional copies of this material (see the box at the end of the Contents).

Circle of Mothers

"I was surprised by how many things feel nourishing to me, even though there are things that I get grouchy about. Sometimes I think I don't want to go to work today or I don't want to stay home with the baby today, but really there's a lot of things that I do at work and at home that are nourishing to me and that I think I enjoy. They can be small pieces of my day, so maybe I don't notice them always, but they do nourish me."

"I was surprised to see how many parts of my day at work are depleting for me. The balance really tips toward depleting. I'm aware of how tired I feel at the end of the day, but I didn't really see that pretty much all of the activities at work are depleting. I realize that I really hate my job. It was almost all depleting activities. This helps me see really clearly—yeah, I really hate my job."

"The waking-up morning time, before we've gotten out of bed, brings a lot of pleasure, but the whole morning routine is one of the things that can be really depleting. I realized writing it down that I'm doing many things at once during the morning. Driving to and from daycare is nourishing because I'm only driving and I can't do anything else. But before then, when I'm trying to do a million things at once to get out the door, that is really depleting."

Pleasure, Mastery, and Connecting Activities

What you do with your time from moment to moment, from hour to hour, from one day to the next, week after week, can have a very powerful influence on your general well-being and your ability to stay well over time. There are three categories of activity that can be particularly helpful in promoting well-being for those who are vulnerable to feeling down, overwhelmed, anxious, or stressed:

1. PLEASURE activities are those that provide a sense of enjoyment.
2. MASTERY activities are those that provide a feeling of accomplishment.
3. CONNECTING activities are those that engage you with other people.

What pleasure, mastery, and connecting activities are a part of your daily routine? You may identify some from your recorded list of nourishing activities and record them in the form on page 142. If you need more space or would like to fill out this form more than once, information on accessing the form online is at the end of the Contents.

The form on page 143 offers some suggestions from the circle of mothers. Circle or highlight any you want to experiment with integrating into your daily routine.

Recognize that pregnancy and parenting may shift how you experience activities. As you examine possible pleasure, mastery, and connecting activities, remember that activities that

My Pleasure, Mastery, and Connecting Activities

Pleasure Activities	Mastery Activities	Connecting Activities

From *Expecting Mindfully: Nourish Your Emotional Well-Being and Prevent Depression during Pregnancy and Postpartum,* by Sona Dimidjian and Sherryl H. Goodman. Copyright © 2019 The Guilford Press. Purchasers of this book can photocopy and/or download additional copies of this material (see the box at the end of the Contents).

used to fit into these categories may shift during pregnancy and parenting. For example, Aisha and her partner loved going out to dinner as a pleasure and a connecting activity before they became parents, but they discovered that going out to dinner with a fussy 3-month-old more often than not was a depleting activity. On the other hand, having the kind of casual dinner at home that might have seemed boring before the baby was born now brought pleasure, mastery, and connection because they divided up the cooking tasks, relaxed in the company of each other and the baby, and left the dishes till the next day.

Thus, experiment with a range of activities and don't limit yourself only to the favorite few that worked for you in the past. It's useful to have a wide range of options, particularly during pregnancy and with a new baby, when some of your old favorites may be harder to do. Also, most moms find that as soon as they become accustomed to a particular stage of parenting, the child changes, and they are in new terrain. For example, Aisha and her partner may well enjoy going out to dinner with their son when he is a few months older. Keeping an open mind and experimenting will help you develop your own broad list of activities that work well specifically for you, even if they shift over time. Also, as we discussed in Class 4, the skills of mindfulness help you stay attuned to the constantly changing nature of experience during pregnancy and postpartum (and life in general!).

Don't Dismiss the Power of Seemingly Small Activities

Often, during pregnancy and early parenting, big activities are just not realistic. The pleasure, mastery, or connecting activities may need to be very small and simple—these might be all that is possible for you to do. For example, when the never-ending laundry is depleting you and you feel a sense of discouragement and hopelessness, be willing to explore small shifts. Maybe you can put on music you love while doing the laundry. Maybe you can stop in the middle and sit down for one single breath. It doesn't sound like a lot, but be willing to experiment with small steps, noticing the possibility of shifting things. Often, the skill is finding small moments of peace, stillness, and self-care in the midst of chaos or stress.

Suggested Pleasure, Mastery, and Connecting Activities from the Circle of Mothers

Pleasure Activities	Mastery Activities	Connecting Activities
Be kind to your body: Sleep or rest (this is critical with a new baby!); nourish yourself with healthy foods; drink plenty of fluids to stay hydrated (especially if you are nursing); take a walk or do another movement activity. *Do something you enjoy:* Do a favorite hobby; cook a meal or snack; go shopping; watch something funny or uplifting on TV; read something that gives you pleasure; practice the lovingkindness meditation; open a gift for the baby; look at photos that give you pleasure. *Engage your senses (even if just for a moment):* Taste a favorite food or drink; smell a scent you enjoy (flowers, perfume, moisturizer, tea); feel the warmth of a shower or bath on your skin; feel the sun or fresh air on your face; listen to your favorite music; watch a sunrise or sunset or another beautiful view.	*Take one step at a time:* Break tasks down into manageable, smaller steps and tackle only *one step at a time* (no more!) to give you a sense of accomplishment. Some examples include doing an exercise class, cooking a new recipe, tackling one item on your to-do list, returning one e-mail or phone call, folding one pile of laundry, unloading the dishwasher. *Acknowledge yourself for taking the step:* For example, instead of setting yourself the task of "paying bills," start with the first step of gathering all the bills into one stack and pause to acknowledge this step as an accomplishment. *Remind yourself that each step you do will build on the others to help you build greater mastery over time:* For example, tell yourself that making the stack of bills will help you get closer to the step of paying them.	*Reach out to other adults:* Spend time with your husband or partner, go on a walk with a friend, talk with a friend or relative on the phone. *Engage with your baby or children:* Take some time to be with your baby or child without trying to accomplish anything or multitask. Play with your baby, watch your child smile, or listen to your child laugh. *Come back to engaging with others when your attention wanders:* For example, "I am picking up my baby; I am feeling my baby's breathing against my chest. . . . Hmm, we need to get more diapers before tonight. . . . I'm noticing that my attention is wandering to planning for the future. I'm coming back to noticing the feeling of my baby breathing. . . . "

Cultivate Awareness of Depleting Activities to Shift Your Relationship to the Ones You Are Stuck With

All of us have certain activities in our days that are depleting. Sometimes these activities can be changed or minimized, and other times they are simply a part of life. For example, on certain days the very thought of another load of laundry was exhausting for Robin. Not doing the laundry was not an option, nor was finding someone else to do it. Sometimes she would avoid the laundry, and it would just pile up. Other times she did it begrudgingly, finding herself more and more irritated and depleted. Robin began to practice the 3-minute coping breathing space when the feelings of exhaustion arose as she looked at the laundry hamper. By bringing awareness to her thoughts, emotions, and sensations in her body, she began to shift her relationship to the activity of laundry. She noted thoughts like "I don't have the energy for this"; "This is never ending"; and "I can't get ahead." She began to be a little friendlier to her experience, acknowledging the ways in which the repetitiveness of laundry with a newborn is challenging without adding on with thoughts that made the experience seem permanent ("never ending") or made her seem to be a failure ("I can't get ahead"). With practice, Robin continued to experience doing the laundry as unpleasant, but it was no longer depleting in the way that it had been.

Make Nourishing Activities Part of Your Routine to Help You Stay Well

Adding pleasure, mastery, and connecting activities as part of your regular schedule, starting now, can be helpful in two ways. First, maintaining these activities in your schedule on a regular basis now can promote your wellness on a daily basis, which can, in turn, help to protect you from depression if you're vulnerable to it. Second, developing a habit of helpful activity now makes it easier to use those activities when you face challenging times, like caring for a new baby or when your mood is low. For example, daily exercise can be very valuable for many people. Daily 10-minute walks or other types of exercise, such as mindful stretching, yoga, swimming, and jogging, can be very helpful for increasing energy and positive mood on a daily basis. Once exercise is in your daily routine, it's more easily available as a response to depressed moods if they arise in the future.

Daily Practice for Lesson 2

Review your list of activities, and for each day this week, plan and commit to doing at least one pleasure, mastery, or connecting activity.

- ◆ Remember that these can be small, simple, and brief. Don't expect miracles from these activities. Instead, carry out what you've planned

> as best you can and remember that you may feel the benefits of some
> activities over time rather than right away.
>
> ◆ Write down these commitments for each day in your Practice Journal on
> the first line of the Lesson 2 Reflection column under "Planned activity."
> Once you've completed the activity, write down what you observed.

Lesson 3. Warning Signs and Action Plans

All moms and moms-to-be have tough times—nights when their baby barely sleeps, days
when they wonder how they can manage everything, moments when they and their partner
argue. If you've experienced depression in the past, these experiences have the potential to
kick off a downward spiral into depression. If you've experienced anxiety, such experiences
may trigger increases in worry, agitation, and stress. The good news is that you can learn to
use these tough times and your responses as information to take care of yourself and be the
most effective mom you can be. The collection of specific situations, thoughts, emotions, and
sensations that indicate that you're at risk are called your "warning signs," and each of us has
our own specific set.

These are the types of reflections that women share with us after they have learned to identify
their own warning signs:

- "I feel tired a lot of the time with the new baby, but when I start to feel a heaviness that
  persists for most of the day, I know I'm at risk for slipping into a depression."

- "Guilt is a big red-flag emotion for me. When it starts to stick around, it's a sign."

- "The thoughts that pop up over and over are the big warning signs for me—especially
  the ones that say 'You're a terrible mother; you can't do anything right.' "

- "I cry a lot and over things that wouldn't typically upset me. Like if my toddler spills
  something at the table, I feel like I'm going to burst into tears."

- "I start to refuse invitations from my friends to get together. I start thinking that it's not
  worth the hassle."

- "I get so irritable with everything and everyone. I tell myself that things are not a big
  deal, but I just feel so annoyed. That is my big clue that things are going off course."

Warning signs can be evident in the body, in emotions, in thoughts, and in actions. In the
form on page 146, we provide examples of warning signs in each of these categories. These
lists are not exhaustive, and what matters most is identifying the warning signs that are most

Noticing and Responding to Warning Signs

Common Warning Signs	My Warning Signs	My Pleasure, Mastery, and Connecting Activities
Warning signs in my body (feeling exhausted, sleeping more or less, eating more or less or different kinds of foods, aches and pains, etc.)		
Warning signs in my emotions (feeling sad, down, guilty, irritable, ashamed, angry, numb, overwhelmed, etc.)		
Warning signs in my thoughts (critical of others, down on myself, etc.)		
Warning signs in my actions (withdrawing from other people, procrastinating on tasks, snapping at others, etc.)		

From *Expecting Mindfully: Nourish Your Emotional Well-Being and Prevent Depression during Pregnancy and Postpartum,* by Sona Dimidjian and Sherryl H. Goodman. Copyright © 2019 The Guilford Press. Purchasers of this book can photocopy and/or download additional copies of this material (see the box at the end of the Contents).

informative for you. On page 146, list what specific warning signs are true for you in the second column. You can ignore the third column for now. If you need more space to fill out the form, see the information on accessing the form online at the end of the Contents.

Taking Action When Warning Signs Are Present

The pleasure, mastery, and connecting activities with which you have been practicing are essential supports when warning signs are present. Doing these activities when you're feeling down, stressed, or overwhelmed can help you care for yourself. In fact, what you need during times of difficulty may be no different from what you've practiced many times throughout this course.

It can be helpful to read about what other moms and moms-to-be have identified as possible activities to care for themselves during tough times. Here are a few warning signs and helpful activities that some mothers have shared with us.

Circle of Mothers

Body Warning Signs and Activities

"My main body warning sign is fatigue. And the main self-care activity is simple: sleep, sleep, and sleep. Not easy, but simple. I have to prioritize sleep over everything else. Talk with my husband about this and remind myself that all other tasks can wait for a few days until I'm more rested."

Emotion Warning Signs and Activities

"Sadness is a big warning sign for me. My main activities to take care of myself are doing things that are gentle and enjoyable: take a bath, listen to music I love, and get physically active. When I'm feeling down, I remind myself to take the baby out for a walk, even a short one, every day."

Thought Warning Signs and Activities

"I start to criticize myself a lot. My main healthy activity is to remind myself that thoughts are not facts. I also need to pull out my list of ways to work with challenging thoughts and practice even just one."

Action Warning Signs and Activities

"Isolating myself is my main warning sign. It's not as much about what I do as what I don't do. So my main activity to take care of myself is to reach out to other people. I need to tell my neighbor that I'm feeling down and ask if we can make a morning coffee date or phone call check-in each day for a while."

Return to the form on page 146 and list some activities in the third column that may be helpful to you if those warning signs were to appear in the future.

*Take a 3-Minute Breathing Space to Guide What to Do Next When You Notice
a Warning Sign*

When noticing any of your warning signs, remember that you can rely on the 3-minute breathing space to guide what action to take. Sometimes taking a breathing space provides the expanded perspective that is all you need to care for yourself in the moment and respond to the warning sign. At other times, additional actions are needed. Take a breathing space and then ask yourself: What do I need to do for myself right now? How can I best take care of myself right now? Can I use one of my pleasure, mastery, or connecting activities? If action is indicated, choose from the list you've created for yourself in the form on page 146.

Daily Practice for Lesson 3

One important way to begin to pull together all of what you've practiced and learned in this class is to write a letter to "yourself in the future." This is a letter from yourself now to yourself at some time in the future, when you may be struggling with stress or low mood. It is one way to give "yourself in the future" some of your hard-earned wisdom that might otherwise be tough to access at that time.

There is no right or wrong way to write such a letter. Let your imagination be your guide!

Some women have:

♦ Written handwritten letters that are organized in the framework we suggest below.

♦ Written checklists that they have called an "operating manual."

♦ Written notes to themselves that they stuck on the bathroom mirror or in the kitchen and other places they frequently go.

♦ Not written a word and instead have created "care packages" or "tool boxes" that contain objects to remind and support them in recognizing warning signs and taking action.

It's critical to remember that these letters are "living documents" and "works in progress." We encourage you to continue to add to them as your awareness of how to care for yourself expands or changes over time.

We invite you to experiment with writing a letter to "yourself in the future." As you begin the letter, you might address the frame of mind that you might be in at the time— for example, "I know you probably will not feel hopeful about this idea, and I know you may be thinking that nothing will help, but trust me, this is really important. . . . " Then you may want to address some of these questions that are linked to the sections we've covered in this chapter:

◆ What are my warning signs that depression may be trying to take hold again? What are the changes that are important for me to be on the lookout for? What are some particular warning signs that might be true for me in late pregnancy or with a new baby?

◆ Who in my life can be part of an "early warning system"? Who can help me be on the lookout for warning signs as I transition to life with my new baby? What steps can I take now to include this person as part of my "early warning system"?

◆ What actions can I take to respond skillfully when my support people or I notice these warning signs?

◆ What would make it hard for me to put these plans into action? What can I do or say to myself now that might make it easier to overcome these obstacles to caring for myself in the future, especially with a new baby?

If it's helpful to you, you can use the form on page 150. Or you can use your own favorite paper, write something online, make a care package, or something else. This week, spend some time each day reflecting on and writing your letter.

Daily Practice Summary

To recap, we invite you to do the following daily practices and record your experiences in your Practice Journal.

Lesson 1

• Practice the lovingkindness meditation each day, using the audio guides to support your practice. You can do either the sitting (Track 15) or walking lovingkindness practice (Track 16). You can alternate between them, do both each day, or choose one for the week. If it's helpful, you also can listen to the "Introduction to Lovingkindness Meditation" (Track 14) again, to remind you of the intention of these practices.

• Briefly record what you notice during your practice in the Practice Journal.

Lesson 2

- Do the pleasure, mastery, or connecting activity that you planned for each day. Again, don't expect miracles from these activities; carry out what you've planned as best you can and remember that you may feel the benefits of some activities over time rather than immediately. Once you've completed the activity, write down what you observed.

Lesson 3

- Write the letter to "yourself in the future." As a first step, please complete the template on the facing page. You can use your completed template as your letter, or you can use it as the foundation for any of the suggestions listed in Lesson 3. Let your imagination be your guide! Spend time each day reflecting on ideas for writing, revising, or reviewing your letter.

Circle of Support:

- On at least one day, talk with your support person about what you learned from this chapter and what you are noticing in your daily practices. Record any reflections based on these conversations in the Circle of Support Reflections.

Letter to Yourself in the Future Template

Dear _____:

I know you probably will not feel hopeful about this idea, and I know you may be thinking that nothing will help, but trust me, this is really important.

If you're reading this, you may be feeling or noticing these experiences in your body, thoughts, emotions, or actions [list here your warning signs]:

Remember that you have people around you who want to be part of looking out for you. Reach out to at least one of these people [list your "early warning system" people here]:

You've worked really hard to identify actions that you can take to respond skillfully when your warning signs are present.

Do yourself a favor and practice with one or two of these activities, even if you don't feel like doing them [list here your pleasure, mastery, connecting activity options]:

I know you're going to have a list of reasons and barriers to doing these activities. I want to remind you of some important wisdom that you developed through this class [list here your reminders of how to make it easier to overcome obstacles to caring for yourself in the future, especially with a new baby]:

Thank you for taking these steps, even though it's hard to do!

Love,

Me

Practice Journal

	Day 1	Day 2	Day 3
Lesson 1 Practice Reflections: What did you notice in your lovingkindness practice today?			
Example: *The sitting lovingkindness meditation was a struggle at the start. It was a challenge for me to concentrate when I was focusing on myself. When I switched my attention to others, I connected more strongly to the phrases. I am curious if over time I will feel similarly when I use the phrases toward myself. It's interesting to notice just how hard it is for me to be loving and kind with myself.*			
Lesson 2 Practice Reflections: Of your planned pleasure, mastery, or connecting activities, what did you do today? In what ways was it nourishing? What did you notice about the balance of nourishing and depleting today?			
Example: *Planned activity: I planned to take a brief nap in the afternoon today as a pleasure activity. I slept for about 30 minutes, and it felt so good!*	Planned activity:	Planned activity:	Planned activity:
Lesson 3 Practice Reflections: Put a check mark on the days in which you worked on your letter.			
Example: ✓			

Practice Journal

Day 4	Day 5	Day 6	Day 7
Planned activity:	Planned activity:	Planned activity:	Planned activity:

Circle of Support Reflections

What did you notice in connecting with your support person this week?

CLASS 7

Expanding Your Circle of Care

Alone we can do so little; together we can do so much.
—Helen Keller

This chapter includes the following three lessons:

1. **Myths about motherhood can make it hard to care for yourself when pregnant and parenting.** We invite you to become aware of myths that may be interfering with caring for yourself and to commit to daily practices that will anchor your growing skills of mindfulness.

2. **The 3-minute breathing space continues to be one of the main tools to support you in responding wisely to challenges and difficulties.** We guide you in a practice called "the four doors" that can be used after taking a 3-minute breathing space to cope with challenge or difficulty.

3. **It really does take a village to be pregnant and care for a baby . . . or, at least, it takes more than just you. All mothers need and deserve help and support.** We invite you to expand the circles of care for you and your baby by practicing specific skills in reaching out to others for support and in saying no when needed.

Lesson 1. Myths about Motherhood

In our last class you explored pleasure, mastery, and connecting activities to bring more nourishing experiences into your day. You also learned practices of lovingkindness in which you held your baby, your family, and yourself in your awareness, establishing an essential foundation in which the love and care of everyone—including you—is connected. As important as these activities are, they often are tough to practice routinely during pregnancy or with a new baby.

155

Part of what makes it hard to practice is the messages about being a mother that we absorb, often without our awareness. These messages come from so many places:

- Stories we hear and see on TV, in movies, and in the news and social media

- Examples of other women we observe in our families and neighborhoods

- Advice and feedback given directly to us by our families, friends, or even strangers

- Information we read online, in magazines, or books

- Guidance or instruction we receive from parenting experts, doctors, and other professionals

- Our own history of experience with asking for help or having others ask us for things

Much of what we have learned can help and support us as we transition to becoming mothers, but sometimes we also absorb myths that we take as truths (with a capital T!) about ourselves or about the world. These myths prescribe what it means to be a mother, what a "good" mother thinks, feels, does, and doesn't do.

You may not think you're impacted by these myths, but you might be surprised by what you discover when you bring mindful attention and curiosity to the myths. As Peg explained: "I didn't think the myths about pregnancy or parenting had much to do with me. I'm pretty clear about my own values. In fact, I often think of myself as disliking or rejecting a lot of common myths about pregnancy and being a mom. As I started to pay closer attention to the myths and reflect on their presence in my life, I saw just how such myths actually are embedded in the ways I think and act about pregnancy. Fortunately, just because they are embedded doesn't mean that they get to control me! Noticing them and making choices with awareness is such a better path."

Bringing these myths into awareness offers us the possibility of greater freedom as we move forward in pregnancy and becoming mothers.

Read the following list and circle the sentences below that are familiar and that function as myths in your life. If this list reminds you of other ideas that are not listed, there is space for you to add them at the bottom.

Remember that what matters is how the idea works in your life. What is a myth for one person might be a valued belief for another, and that's perfectly fine. The point is to bring awareness to whether these beliefs are part of your core values or represent inherited or adopted beliefs that don't feel right for you or interfere with your well-being, parenting, or other aspects of your family life.

1. It's not okay to want or need something from someone else.
2. A good mother is strong but not too strong, assertive but not overbearing.
3. A good mother should be willing to sacrifice her own needs for others.
4. It's okay to ask for something for my baby but not for myself.
5. I should be able to handle being pregnant and taking care of a baby on my own.
6. Doing things for yourself or asking other people for help is selfish.
7. Good mothers don't get overwhelmed (e.g., get angry, "lose it," cry, feel unhappy).
8. It's important that I please and support others all the time.
9. If I ask others for help, they will know that I don't know what I'm doing.
10. If I ask others for help, I will be burdening them.
11. I'm the only one who can't handle all this on my own.
12. I can't ask for something if it will inconvenience other people.
13. If other people really cared, they would know what I need without my having to ask for it.
14. If someone says no to my request, it means that I shouldn't have asked or that it was bad to ask in the first place.
15. It's selfish to say no to other people's requests.
16. Saying no to other people will make them think that I don't like or care about them.
17. I can't feel at ease if someone else is frustrated with me for saying no.
18. I am not worthy or good enough to get what I want.
19. Other people have problems of their own; I shouldn't burden them with mine.
20. It's not fair that I have to tell people what I need; it should be obvious.
21. Other: _____
22. Other: _____
23. Other: _____
24. Other: _____

Practice Now

It's not always easy to tell whether an idea you've heard (either growing up or as an adult) is a myth that you don't truly believe in your heart of hearts or has become a value you hold dear. That's where practice comes in.

Let's practice now. Please bring to mind a recent situation in which you felt isolated, alone, stressed, or overwhelmed. Select a situation that is difficult—although not the most difficult thing you can imagine. Perhaps consider a situation that is about a 3 on a difficulty scale of 0 (not difficult at all) to 10 (the most difficult ever). Take a few moments to recall the situation, imagining it in full detail.

Briefly describe the situation: what happened and what was tough about the situation for you?

_____

_____

_____

_____

Now, reviewing the list of myths above, can you identify any myths that might have popped into your mind or that might have been lurking in the back of your awareness during or after the situation you described:

_____

_____

_____

_____

In what ways might the myths have influenced how you felt and what you did (even if you weren't aware of it at the time)?

_____

_____

_____

_____

As you reflect on your vision for staying well during pregnancy, postpartum, and beyond, how might identifying myths, even after the situation has occurred, support you along the staying-well path?

_____

_____

_____

_____

Circle
of Mothers

"My situation was a recent time that I was in the checkout line at the grocery store when I was pregnant. As I was putting my favorite snacks on the belt, the woman behind me leaned over to say, 'You've got to watch what you eat now; you should be eating for that baby more than yourself.' I couldn't believe that she felt free to talk to me like that. I can still feel how my face flushed, and I felt so embarrassed. And even now, her comment has stayed with me. I wonder if I'm a bad mom, wanting things that feel good to me without always thinking first if it's good for the baby. I realize that is one of the myths, and it definitely was there and part of how embarrassed I felt in the moment . . . and the insecure feeling that lingered. When I reflect on this, I realize that the belief that it's not okay for me to have what I want in my life and that I should always and only think of the baby is not a value I hold dear. In fact, that kind of thinking will get me into trouble because it sets me up to be depleted and at risk of getting depressed."

"What came to mind for me was how I felt annoyed about an e-mail I got from my son's school about volunteering for the class play. I know it's on the 'myth list,' but I do believe that saying no to other people is selfish. It's not a myth for me; it's a value I hold dear. I am always so amazed at how many other people say no to things that are really important, like volunteering in the classroom or with events at school. My son's teacher really needs the help, so I said yes, even though it means juggling things with the baby. This practice helped me realize that I can feel good about saying yes to others because I value being generous and giving."

"My situation was kind of a regular thing for me with three kids: how I respond when one of my kids is sick. Especially in the winter, it seems like someone is always sick. I think that I absorbed multiple messages from watching my mom take care of me and my brothers. Watching her do everything she did as a single mom, I definitely learned about being strong and capable. I think that's helped me a lot. But I think I also absorbed some lessons about other people being unreliable or its being better to just take care of things yourself. Sometimes I realize that I don't even think of asking for help because of that, and I put a lot of unnecessary pressure on myself as a result. Immediately, I am trying to figure out how I can do it all with work and the other kids and taking care of the one who is sick. I have great friends, and my husband wants to be supportive; I just don't reach out to them. I don't even think of it as an option most times. Recognizing this myth and all the extra stress and strain it has caused me—that has helped to give me more choices in the moment."

Daily Practice for Lesson 1

Identifying the myths provides an opportunity to get curious about them, just as we did with thoughts in Class 5. Yet, it's hard work. One of the key lessons of this chapter is that these myths are insidious—we have gotten so used to them coming from others, or they are such a part of our cultural background (or both), that it takes well-developed mindfulness to become aware of when they are "on the scene." They might pop into your mind or be hovering in the background without your awareness.

Maintaining daily formal and informal mindfulness practice is an excellent way to continue developing your skill at recognizing and observing thoughts, and this provides a great foundation for working directly with myths. Rather than getting ambushed or carried away by the myths in ways that affect your mood and behavior, a little daily mindfulness practice, over time, can strengthen your awareness and capacity to make choices that support your well-being. We explore a practice directly focused on the myths following Lesson 3; for now, though, we invite you to select *one formal and one informal mindfulness practice* from all the ones that you have learned—practices that will be truly yours in the weeks to come.

◆ Take a moment to read over the list of formal practices below. Select one that you intend to use on a regular basis after you complete this eight-class series. You might consider making a daily commitment to one of these practices for, say, a month after you complete the eight-class series. After that month, you can return and select another if you wish; for now, though, identify one on which you can rely as an anchor for your growing skills of mindfulness.

- The body scan (page 30)
- 10-minute sitting meditation (page 53)
- 25-minute sitting meditation (page 63)
- Yoga (page 67)
- Walking meditation (page 68)
- 3-minute breathing space (scheduled at routine times during the day) (page 77)
- Lovingkindness sitting meditation (page 133)
- Lovingkindness walking meditation (page 133)

◆ Now take a moment to read over the list of daily activities below that you can use for informal practice. We invite you to settle on one activity to use for your *informal daily practice* on a regular basis after you complete this eight-class series. Again, you might consider making a daily commitment to the practice you select for, say, a month after you complete the eight-class series. After that month you can return and select another if you wish; for now, though, committing to one daily informal practice will increase the likelihood of your remembering to do it and making it a part of your daily routine.

- Being with your baby
- Checking e-mail or text messages
- Listening to music
- Cooking
- Waking up in the morning
- Saying good morning/good night
- Getting into bed at night
- Using the phone
- Folding laundry
- Washing dishes
- Settling into a meeting at work
- Sweeping floors
- Scrubbing tubs, floors, toilets
- Straightening up
- Taking out the garbage
- Driving
- Waiting in line
- Brushing teeth, bathing, showering
- Getting dressed
- Brushing/drying hair
- Other: _____

◆ Practice the formal and informal practices you selected each day this week. Briefly record what you notice during your practice in your Practice Journal.

Lesson 2. Using the "Four Doors"

Catching when myths about motherhood are present is critical to preventing the myths from influencing how we feel or what we do. Sometimes, though, awareness is not enough.

Anya struggled with intense exhaustion when her baby was a few weeks old: "I had this expectation that things would be pretty peaceful when the baby came. Like, lots of afternoons of nursing on the glider, sort of admiring how amazing he is. Don't get me wrong, he is amazing and I love him, but there are not a lot of peaceful moments. He's super fussy, and we rarely sit down. He needs to be constantly walked, changed, and his feedings are short and frequent. I'm exhausted. It's intense parenting 100% of the time, and I keep thinking that I should be able to handle this. My sister-in-law has three kids and doesn't seem to be crushed by it. I can see that I'm being ruled by some myths—like If I ask others for help, they will know that I'm not a good mother. When I have that thought, I just feel worse and I pull away from my husband and friends . . . I can see all of this, but I'm not sure what to do about it. I'm still exhausted."

Anya is relying on her skills of mindfulness to recognize her strong emotions and physical exhaustion. She also sees the myths that are present and how they are impacting her. And yet, what is Anya to do in such a situation?

What can you do when you notice the myths are in full force and you're overwhelmed?

The 3-minute breathing space is always the first step: acknowledging your experience, gathering your attention at the breath, and then expanding back to your thoughts, emotions, and body.

Sometimes the simple practice of bringing attention helps to shift experience. Recall in the last chapter when we explored how you might find some moments of peace in the unlikeliest of activities—feeling depleted by daily loads of laundry. This was a frequent occurrence for Robin. She struggled with never being finished with laundry and experienced a strong sense of discouragement and hopelessness. Myths of motherhood were, indeed, in full force: "I should be able to handle this on my own. My partner should care enough about me to know what I need without my having to ask for it. Isn't it obvious from the piles of laundry in the hallway?" In the breathing space, she felt more willing to open to the reality that the laundry and feelings of frustration are part of the flux and flow of daily life when caring for a new baby. For Robin, this expanded awareness and acceptance was enough to reengage with a greater sense of balance.

Sometimes, though, the breathing space indicates that more is required. As Anya experienced, "I've felt lost in noticing all that is challenging and just feeling overwhelmed, even after I finish the breathing space. In these moments, I want something structured to guide me in what to do next."

Following the 3-minute breathing space with a practice called the "four doors" can provide just the guidance that Anya was seeking. These four doors provide options or openings through which you have the choice to walk. The four doors available to you are:

1. *The reentry door*: This option invites you to shift your experience by expanding your awareness, as in the laundry example. You can reenter the same experience with a different relationship to the challenges, one that is a little friendlier, open, and allowing.

2. *The body door*: This option invites you to bring awareness to the ways in which distressing situations manifest as sensations in the body, noticing tension, aching, and/or tightness. As you attend and open to these sensations, you may find it easier to let go than to struggle with them.

3. *The thought door*: This option invites you to notice ways in which you may be adding on thoughts that are making the situation harder. You may find, in particular, that problems are compounded by thoughts about being a mom, asking other people for help, or saying no to other people's requests or expectations of you. Entering the "thought door" asks you to bring awareness to these thoughts and the influence that they may be having on your experience. You might ask yourself, "Am I confusing a myth with a fact?" Or remind yourself that myths are just that—myths—perhaps, gently noting, "A lot of mothers have these thoughts; they are not specific to me; they are not truth with a capital T."

4. *The action door*: This option invites you to consider taking wise action. For women who are pregnant or parenting, the action often involves taking small steps, such as using a pleasure, mastery, or connecting activity in the small moments of daily life (e.g., listening to a podcast while doing the laundry, pausing after closing the washer door to pay attention to one single exhale, etc.). These actions may not seem like a lot, but it's important to be willing to experiment with them and discover whether your experience shifts. These small actions can create brief moments of peace, stillness, and self-care in the midst of chaos or unending demands. Doing so, though, often requires practicing an action that is relevant for many women during pregnancy and parenting—the wise action of asking for help and saying no. We explore this more in Lesson 3.

Practice Now

Using the 3-minute breathing space and the "four doors," we invite you to practice now with a situation in which you felt overwhelmed, stressed, or down (and perhaps myths were present). Bring a situation to mind that is not the most difficult thing you can imagine, about a 3 on a difficulty scale of 0 (not difficult at all) to 10 (the most difficult ever).

Practice the steps of the 3-minute breathing space, supported by listening to audio Track 10, "3-Minute Breathing Space," if you wish, and when you've completed the third step, reflect on which of the four doors would be most helpful to you:

◆ Reentry Door

◆ Body Door

◆ Thought Door

◆ Action Door

When you're finished, please return to reflect on your experience.

Reflections on Practice

What did you notice in your experience of the 3-minute breathing space?

_____

_____

_____

_____

Which of the four doors did you find the most helpful and supportive for you in responding to the difficult situation you brought to mind? How was it helpful?

_____

_____

_____

_____

As you reflect on your vision for staying well during pregnancy, postpartum, and beyond, how might this practice support you along the staying-well path?

_____

_____

_____

_____

Women in the circle of mothers described the many benefits that they experienced learning to use the 3-minute breathing space in routine moments of the day in Class 3 and to cope with difficult situations in Class 4. Here they continue to describe ways in which expanding their practice of the 3-minute breathing space with the "four doors" has been helpful.

Circle of Mothers

"The body door was really helpful for me. I noticed that my shoulders had loosened a bit, but there was still so much tension in my body. I spent a few more minutes allowing myself to let go of some of that tightness as I exhaled. I focused a lot on my shoulders and neck, and also my hands, which I realized I was clenching."

"The thought door is a big one that I use a lot. I often have to walk through that in order to cope with the situations I find myself in. With this one, I noticed that I was adding on a lot of thoughts about how I don't know what I'm doing. I realize that I feel worse the more I tell myself that. So, when I walk through the 'thought door,' I remind myself to ask, 'Am I confusing a thought with a fact here?' More often than not, the answer is yes."

"Taking the breathing space helps me pause, and just breathing itself is helpful to give me a moment to calm down. As I've done a few breathing spaces when the baby is fussy, though, I've realized that I'm in the same situation over and over recently. So, this time, the image of the four doors really helped. I thought, I can walk through that action door. I can do something. I decided that I will call our pediatrician and talk over things with the nurse about what's been happening. Maybe she will have some ideas about what I can do to help soothe him if he gets worked up like that in the future."

Daily Practice for Lesson 2

This week we invite you to build on the imaginal practice you just completed.

- Use the coping 3-minute breathing space and the "four doors" as difficult situations arise in your daily life. Record the number of times you practice by circling "Coping 3MBS."

- Additionally, record in your Practice Journal what you notice in using the 3-minute breathing space and the "four doors" practice.

- You may use the guided instructions (Track 10), or you can review the instructions for the coping 3MBS on page 97.

Lesson 3. Asking for Help and Saying No

For many women, maintaining a healthy balance of nourishing and depleting activities during pregnancy and parenting requires expanding the circle of care. This might mean bringing new people into your life who can support you, reducing time or contact with people in your life who don't support you, or engaging the people already in your life to support you in the ways you find most valuable. In all of these cases, asking for help and saying no to other people's requests or demands on your time are critical skills. Engaging the assistance and support of other people enables you to maintain the activities that help you stay well and restore balance to what nourishes you.

As a starting point, let's explore how easy or difficult it is to ask for what you want or to say no to other people's requests or demands on your time.

What is your experience of asking other people for help? Put an "X" on the line where you locate yourself on the range of ease/challenge of asking for help:

1 _____ 10

No problem; it's easy!   Impossible; I can't imagine!

What is your experience of saying no to other people's requests? Put an "X" on the line where you locate yourself on the range of ease/challenge of saying no to others' requests:

1 _____ 10

No problem; it's easy!   Impossible; I can't imagine!

For many, asking for help or saying no to other people's requests is difficult. Even if you're generally skillful at asking for help or saying no, your skills can be challenged during pregnancy and postpartum. The combination of all the biological changes in your body, the lack of sleep, and other challenges can make it hard to access skills that came easily at other times in your life. Also, even though you may have very supportive relationships in your life, being pregnant and having a baby can put added stress on these relationships in ways that require even greater skill in asking for help and saying no.

The good news is that, like all the other skills we've practiced, mindfully asking for help and saying no are skills that can be learned and strengthened over time with practice. We can begin to practice directly asking for help and saying no by using four simple questions to help us determine exactly what we want to say:

1. What is the situation?

2. How do I feel about it?

3. What do I want?

4. What are the benefits of agreeing to what I am asking?

These questions are based on an interpersonal effectiveness skill developed by our friend and colleague Marsha Linehan that has helped thousands of people ask for the help they need or say no to requests from others. When we ask ourselves the questions, it's important to stick to the facts of the situation and clearly state how we feel about it, what we need, and what the positive consequences of agreeing to our wishes will be (or the negative consequences of denying our wishes).

Once we have a simple script in mind (or on paper if preferred), we need to prepare for how to deliver the message: staying mindful during the conversation, demonstrating confidence, and conveying our openness to negotiating. Here are some tips to keep in mind:

- Keep your focus on your goals.

- Maintain your position.

- Avoid distraction.

- Stay on topic.

- Be a "broken record" if needed: Keep asking, saying no, or expressing your opinion over and over. Just keep restating the same thing again and again.

- Ignore any threats, comments, or attempts to change the subject.

- Adopt a confident tone of voice and physical manner, with good eye contact, even if you don't feel confident in the moment.

- Avoid stammering, whispering, staring at the floor, retreating, expressing doubt ("I'm not sure"), or over apologizing ("I'm so sorry to ask this").

- Be willing to give to get: Say no but offer to do something else or to solve the problem another way. Or ask for other solutions to the problem.

- Compromise without giving in: Reduce your request or ask the other person for some possible solutions.

- Focus on the benefits for you and the other person.

How does this work in practice? Let's first consider an example of asking for help. Elaine expected things to be tough after her mother-in-law left. It hadn't been a piece of cake to have her stay with them for the first month since the baby was born, but her mother-in-law had helped so much with errands and cooking. A lot of women in her lactation group would be willing to help, but Elaine couldn't imagine asking them. She started by thinking through the four questions and writing down her answers to come up with what she would say to one of her lactation group friends.

Elaine struggled a bit to come up with a simple statement of her situation because she was feeling so overwhelmed by the number of tasks before her and her guilt over asking for help. Using mindfulness, she zeroed in on meals as being a big issue for her and also recognized the fear she felt that she wouldn't be able to manage without her mother-in-law. Focusing like this made it easier for her to describe how much the favor she was asking for would help her and how she could eventually reciprocate. Here's what she said:

1. **What is the situation?** "My mother-in-law has been cooking for us for the last few weeks, and she is leaving next Monday. I still am learning the basics of caring for the baby. I don't think I'll have time or energy for cooking a lot of meals when she leaves."

2. **How do I feel about it?** "I feel scared that I won't have the energy to care for my baby if I'm doing other things like cooking, and I'm afraid that I won't eat and then breastfeeding will be even harder because I won't be hydrated or nourished."

3. **What do I want?** "Would you consider bringing over dinner one night a week during the first month after my mother-in-law leaves?"

4. **What are the benefits of agreeing to what I am asking?** "This would help me so much! Our lactation group is so amazing, and you've been such a great friend. I just know that it will make a big difference for me and the baby, and as soon as I get the hang of this mothering thing, I will offer to make a meal for someone else in the group!"

In her practice, Elaine noticed that she kept adding things like "It's totally fine if you can't do it; I understand it's asking a lot" to the end of her request. So she thought about alternatives she could have ready to offer to avoid leaping in with apologies for even asking—willingness to go with whatever night of the week worked for her friend, accept something simple, even be happy with inexpensive takeout. She also committed to staying mindful of how her friend responded so she wouldn't allow her automatic pilot to push her into jumping in with "It's not a big deal if it's doesn't work for you" before her friend even finished a sentence.

Now let's consider an example of saying no. Nella was exhausted at the end of her pregnancy. She was up for most of the night with the baby kicking so much or having to go to the bathroom. The afternoons were the hardest, and her boss had agreed to change her schedule so she had only the morning shift. When another coworker quit, however, he asked her to start covering the afternoons too. Nella was about to say yes and then remembered the four questions.

She worked through each one, avoiding the "kitchen-sinking" of describing her boss's unfairness and the disorganization of the office in her initial statement. Exhaustion made it challenging to sort through her feelings, but as she focused on sensations in her body, a skill she developed through the body scan and sitting meditation practices, she became aware of fear. She was afraid of the impact of expanding her schedule at work. What she needed to ask for—or, in this case, to say no to—was pretty obvious. In reminding her boss of why her request was valid, she decided to stick to how keeping her morning-only schedule would benefit him and the office in general. Here's what she said:

1. **What is the situation?** "We agreed to my working morning shifts only."

2. **How do I feel about it?** "I'm worried about what's going to happen with my schedule."

3. **What do I want?** "It is not possible for me to change my schedule."

4. **What are the benefits of agreeing to what I am asking?** "Keeping my schedule will let me continue to make good contributions in the morning and make it possible for me to keep working until the baby is born. I love my job and want to be part of this team for a long time. Keeping my schedule as it is will make that possible. I would really appreciate your understanding and finding another solution to the afternoon problem."

For Nella, being able to speak to her boss with self-confidence was really important. The first few times she practiced, she tended to look down and away and use a really quiet tone. She realized that if she didn't go into the conversation with more confidence in saying no, he was likely to dwell on how she was the best person for the afternoon. She practiced speaking clearly, making eye contact, and repeating, if needed, "It's not possible for me to change my schedule now." She also committed to staying mindful while she was talking with him and made a plan to tell him she needed to use the restroom for a minute so that she could take a break from the conversation if she started to feel flustered or was considering saying yes instead of no.

If asking for help like Elaine and saying no like Nella sound challenging to you, know that these are skills that develop with practice. Each time you ask for what would help you and each time you say no, you strengthen the skill, and it gets easier to use the next time.

One way to practice is to prepare ahead with tough situations, just as Elaine and Nella did with the friend and the boss. Often these tough situations also are ones where myths are present, telling you that it's not okay to ask for what you want or to say no. In these cases it can be helpful to reflect on and write out your answers to the four questions in advance. Then it can be helpful to practice saying each part out loud before you speak to the other person directly.

Practice Now

Let's practice with the situation that you described above on page 157, in Lesson 1, as you reflected on the presence and impact of myths. Imagine if a similar situation were to occur in the future. Or, if you prefer, you may select a different situation. Use the four steps framework to write out and practice in advance what to say and how to say it.

1. What is the situation?

Describe the current situation. Stick to the facts.

_____

_____

_____

_____

2. How do I feel about it?

Express your feelings and opinions about the situation. Don't assume that the other person knows how you feel.

_____

_____

_____

_____

3. What do I want?

Ask for what you want or say no clearly.

_____

_____

_____

_____

4. What are the benefits of agreeing to what I am asking?

Explain the positive effects of getting what you want or need. If necessary, also clarify the negative consequences of not getting what you want or need.

_____

_____

_____

_____

These questions and ways of speaking mindfully, confidently, and with an openness to negotiating are designed to help you take action to maintain a healthy balance of nourishing and depleting activities and respond to warning signs.

Nourishing activities—like sleeping, taking a shower, or eating a snack—that were routine in the past may be challenging to accomplish when you're pregnant or parenting, even though these activities are essential. As simple as they seem, doing these activities can require the help of others when you're pregnant or caring for a new baby.

Practice Now

Read over the two examples provided in the table below to see how one mom practiced (1) asking for help to get more sleep and (2) saying no to a visit from a friend. Next, use the form on page 172 to identify a few actions that you can take now to help address challenges with the balance of nourishing and depleting activities in your daily life or activities that will become more difficult to do over time.

Examples of How to Practice
Asking for Help and Saying No

What is the challenge?	Who can help?	What do I want or what don't I want?	What action can I take using the four questions to talk with people in my life?
My sleep is out of balance; I'm really depleted from not getting quality sleep	Husband	I want my husband to take the baby for a walk on Saturday mornings so that I can sleep or at least rest.	Remind myself that I'm experiencing "myth thinking," expecting him to know what I want without my saying it and instead planned out what to say tonight to ask for his help.
I'm depleted by so many social events and so much time with other people	Friend and sister	I don't want my friend to stay with us when she visits this weekend; having to hang out and talk with her sounds exhausting when what I really want is some quiet time at home.	Remind myself that I don't want to live by the myth that it's not okay to say no. Ask my sister if my friend can stay at her house; used my answers to the four questions to explain the situation to my friend and say no clearly.

My Plans for Practicing Asking for Help and Saying No

What is the challenge?	Who can help?	What do I want or what don't I want?	What action can I take to talk with people in my life?

From *Expecting Mindfully: Nourish Your Emotional Well-Being and Prevent Depression during Pregnancy and Postpartum,* by Sona Dimidjian and Sherryl H. Goodman. Copyright © 2019 The Guilford Press. Purchasers of this book can photocopy and/or download additional copies of this material (see the box at the end of the Contents).

Fill in the form with at least one example in your own life of how asking for help or saying no can address a challenge with the balance of nourishing and depleting activities. (If you need more space, information about downloading and printing the form are at the end of the Contents.)

1. Identify the challenge that is making it hard to maintain a healthy balance between nourishing and depleting activities in your daily life.

2. Identify who can help. If it's useful, you can refer to the Circles of Connection that you completed in the Getting Started chapter. Who in your Circles of Connection might you call on now? Or are there other people in your life now that you can add to your Circles of Connection?

3. Clarify what you want or what you don't want.

4. Identify some specific actions that you can take, using the four questions as a guide for communicating what you want or don't want to the people in your life.

The four questions also can help in the face of your warning signs and when depression is beginning to take hold. How can you rely on the wisdom of asking yourself these questions at such times? Let's consider the example of Janine, who described experiencing many of her warning signs of depression's return.

Janine said: "I started to feel really overwhelmed, and I was just camping out on the couch and watching things on TV that I'd never watch. It's like I just wanted to escape. It got really hard to even imagine calling someone and saying 'Hey, want to come over for a cup of tea? It would be nice to see you.' I honestly didn't want to do anything. I just had a 'What's the point?' attitude. I would think 'Why don't you call your friend, or why don't you make an appointment with your therapist?' But then, it was like 'What's that going to do?' Plus, I felt embarrassed about the fact that I was kind of hiding out . . . I avoided the stuff that I know helps. I wasn't eating much, wasn't exercising, wasn't talking with friends, stayed up really late watching TV, and was exhausted."

Janine identified a number of warning signs that were present and noticed that some major myths were getting in the way of her taking action. In particular, the myth that it was not okay to ask for help was increasing her sense of shame and urge to hide out. Janine countered these forces with answering the four questions to reach out. Using these, she made a call and left a voicemail for her therapist, even when all she really wanted to do was watch TV on the couch. Here's what she said:

1. What is the situation?

"Hi, it's Janine. I'm calling because I've been starting to have a hard time and I just don't want to do anything or see anyone."

2. How do I feel about it?

"I feel exhausted and awful."

3. What do I want?

"I was wondering if we could talk by phone or maybe if I could come in for a session."

4. What are the benefits of agreeing to what I am asking?

"I think it might help, and I'd really appreciate it if you could call me back."

Janine also kept in mind the focus on *appearing confident.* In the past, she would have added, "It's not a problem if you don't have time to call me back," so she practiced ending the call with saying "Thank you so much for taking my call. I look forward to talking soon." Because she also felt ashamed of having a hard time, she knew that she was vulnerable to downplaying how she felt. She decided to be on the lookout for saying things that minimized the ways in which she was struggling. She also planned to **negotiate** by offering to talk at a time that was convenient for her therapist. Finally, she stayed **mindful** of her experience during the call. She felt the jitteriness in her hands as she made the call, the tension in her neck and shoulders as she listened to her therapist's outgoing message, and the relief she experienced when she finished her message, knowing she had taken an important step.

Daily Practice for Lesson 3

◆ Each day, identify one example of a myth. It's hard work to identify myths in part because we have grown so accustomed to them in our lives. Get curious about the myths, seeing if you can identify any in messages from other people, movies or TV, or in your own thoughts. When you do, make a note in your Practice Journal.

◆ Then experiment with answering the four questions to see if they help you respond more effectively to a situation in which a myth is "on the scene." At least two times this week, practice asking for help or saying no to something that the myth might tell you otherwise not to. This might be something very small, like asking your partner to help with the dishes after dinner, or it might be something more substantial, like asking your boss for time off from work or telling your neighbor that you don't want her to stop by unannounced.

If you struggle with this practice, know that the skills of asking for help and saying no will get stronger with regular, sustained practice.

◆ In addition, we invite you to return to your letter and make any edits that are informed by what you learned from this class. Are there myths that are important to address directly in your letter? Can you include the use of the 3-minute breathing space in more specific ways? Are there new actions that you identified as you reflected on asking for help and saying no that might help you in the future? Did you experience new wisdom from today's class about how to approach the balance of nourishing and depleting activities and how to respond to warning signs?

Daily Practice Summary

To recap, we invite you to do the following daily practices and record your experiences in your Practice Journal.

Lesson 1

- Each day, do the formal and informal mindfulness practices you selected as your anchors once you complete the eight-class series. These will be your main practices once you end the eight-class series. Briefly record what you notice during your practice in your Practice Journal.

Lesson 2

- Each day, take a 3-minute breathing space and use the "four doors" during challenges. Briefly record what you notice during your practice in your Practice Journal.

Lesson 3

- Each day, identify one example of a myth. Record the myth in your Practice Journal.

- Use your answers to the four questions at least two times this week to practice asking for help and saying no, experimenting, in particular, with situations in which myths are present. Briefly record what you notice during your practice in your Practice Journal.

- Use what you learned from asking for help or saying no and the other lessons of this chapter to revise your letter.

Circle of Support

- Share your letter with your support person or other key people in your life. We invite you to read it aloud to this person or these people. Listen to their responses, ideas, and questions. Then ask if they would be willing to be part of your support team after the eight-class series is completed. Ask if they will be part of your "early warning system"—to be on the lookout for signs you may be struggling or vulnerable. Ask if they will be part of your "action plan," so that you can best care for yourself on a routine basis and if the "warning signs" become apparent. Record any reflections based on this conversation in your Circle of Support Reflections.

Practice Journal

	Day 1	Day 2	Day 3
Lesson 1 Practice Reflections: What did you notice in your daily formal and informal mindfulness practice?			
Example: *I picked the yoga for my daily practice because movement is so important for me. I noticed that I felt grateful to be moving, even though I also still notice those critical thoughts about not being at the level that I was before I got pregnant. I also did the "being with baby" and focused on the little sounds she makes when I'm feeding her.*			
Lesson 2 Practice Reflections: What did you notice in using the 3-minute breathing space and the "four doors" practice?			
Example: *I did multiple breathing spaces today, and I noticed that I walked through the thought door a lot! I routinely add on thoughts to already difficult situations, which, of course, makes me feel worse. Reminding myself that "thoughts are not facts" is a lifesaver!*			
Lesson 3 Practice Reflections: What myth did you encounter? Record brief notes about what you said and what you learned on the days you practiced asking for help or saying no in response to a situation in which a myth is "on the scene." Put a check mark on the days in which you revised your letter.			
Example: ✓ *I have been noticing the myth that "I should be able to handle this on my own." It's been so hot lately that I haven't wanted to take the baby out, even though walking is really important for my mood and well-being. I realized I could use the four questions to ask my mom to come help with the baby. When I called her, I focused on how much daily walks benefit me and the baby, and I was clear why I felt uncomfortable taking the baby out in this heat. She agreed to come over, and we made a plan for tomorrow.*			

Practice Journal

Day 4	Day 5	Day 6	Day 7

Circle of Support Reflections

What was your experience sharing your letter with you support person? What did you learn? What did you plan to help you stay well now and in the future?

CLASS 8

Looking to the Future

How we spend our days is, of course, how we spend our lives.

—Annie Dillard

As we arrive at the last class on this journey together, we offer the following three lessons that are intended to support you not only in the coming week but for weeks, months, and years to come:

1. **As you end this course, it can be helpful to reflect on what you've learned.** We begin today with our very first formal mindfulness practice, the body scan, as a reminder of how far we've come over these eight classes.

2. **Anticipating the inevitable challenges can help keep you on track in the future.** We encourage you to consider the nature and frequency of challenges you've already encountered and any potential barriers to practice you could run into in the future and offer strategies for working skillfully with them.

3. **The hopes and dreams that you hold for yourself and your family are a valuable source of power and guidance.** We close with inviting you to reflect on your motivation to continue a daily mindfulness practice to sustain a lifetime of caring for yourself and your child or children.

Lesson 1. Coming Full Circle

The body scan was the first formal mindfulness practice that you learned, in our very first class together. Today we return to this practice.

When you read this invitation to return to the body scan, you may have had immediate associations or memories based on your experience with this practice at the start of the course. Mindfulness practice invites us to notice those expectations without getting caught by them, so that we remain open to whatever arises.

One mother reflected on both her expectations and her surprise: "I've been getting up so early these past few days; I have been so exhausted. When you said we would do the body scan, I had a sense of dread, remembering too what it was like when we started the classes. I thought, I'll never be able to stay awake for this today. But it was just the opposite. I feel more awake now after the practice than I did at the start."

In this way, the practice teaches us that we can start with one idea and then discover something quite different and new. Perhaps ask yourself, "Is there some value for me in practicing being open to and allowing experience, whatever my expectations?" We invite you to approach this body scan practice with a sense of newness and curiosity about what you will discover today.

Practice Now

Take a few moments to prepare your space. Remember that your body today, with all the changes you have experienced, may benefit from different supports than were needed when we began many weeks ago. In fact, the body you explore today is likely to be very different than it was 8 weeks ago, or whenever you began this series of classes. Find a position in which you are relaxed and supported.

When you're ready, listen to Track 5, "The Body Scan," to do the body scan practice now. When you're finished, please return to reflect on your experience.

Reflections on Practice

What sensations did you notice while doing the body scan?

_____

_____

_____

_____

_____

In what ways did the experience of paying attention to your body in this practice, today, differ from your recollection of practicing the body scan at the start of the course?

_____

_____

_____

_____

As you reflect on your vision for staying well during pregnancy, postpartum, and beyond, how might this practice support you along the staying-well path?

_____

_____

_____

_____

Being Open, Curious, and Allowing

Mindfulness practice invites us to be open and curious about whatever we discover in our experience. As you well know from your own experience, so many intense sensations and states are present during pregnancy and early parenting. You likely find some moments delightful—the fluttery movements of the baby growing within, the warmth of embrace with your newborn, and/or the gentle touch of someone who cares for you. And other moments not so much—discomfort in the back, tightness in the belly, feelings of nausea, exhaustion. During the body scan, many of these sensations also arise. On automatic pilot, it's common to react to difficult experiences by pushing them away, getting stuck, or dwelling on them. Also, on automatic pilot, it's easy to miss the pleasant experiences, particularly the brief and fleeting ones. The body scan and all the other mindfulness practices invite you to be willing to open to all your experiences, as they unfold and change, allowing them, even inviting them, into your awareness with a sense of friendliness and curiosity. These skills of being open, curious, and allowing offer an alternative to simply reacting by avoiding or getting stuck in the difficult experiences.

As one mother described: "I felt a lot of pressure in my lower back. It was really intense, but it wasn't necessarily painful. It was interesting, because in the early classes I remember moving around and being fidgety during the body scan to try to be more comfortable. Today I was okay with it even though it was uncomfortable. I felt more at ease."

This expressed a key shift in understanding and experience—it was possible to have intense sensation without its being painful or distressing or struggling against it, as well as intense emotions, which are inevitable aspects of the experience of pregnancy and parenting. Through her practice of the body scan, this mom gave herself the gift of paying attention to the fullness of the journey of pregnancy and parenting as she experienced it moment by moment.

Returning to the body scan also allows us to consider the full arc of learning that has occurred since Class 1. Reflecting on what you've learned from the classes and your daily practice is helpful both in consolidating what you learned and in creating a stepping stone to help you carry such learning into the future. Take a moment to answer the following question.

> *On a scale of 0 ("not at all important") to 10 ("extremely important"), how important has this program been to you? _____ (0–10)*
>
> Please say why you've given this rating.

_____

_____

_____

_____

Other women in our classes have described the ways in which their learning has been important to them as listed in the table on page 183. Take some time now to reflect on what these mothers have shared (first column) and note (second column) the extent to which any of these are present for you and in what ways. If you've experienced other types of changes, you can add those in the blank rows at the end of the table. (Information on printing and downloading the form is available at the end of the Contents if you need more space.)

Lesson 2. Preparing for a Lifetime of Practice as a Mom

To support you in sustaining your practice after our eight classes are completed, we invite you to consider what type and frequency of practice will be most helpful for you and what are potential barriers to practice—and how you can work skillfully with them.

What Type and Frequency of Practice Will Be Most Helpful For Me?

Settling on a daily practice to continue after the weekly classes end invites you to commit to time for yourself each day. This can be hard when schedules are busy, when demands increase as you prepare for your baby's arrival, and in the early months *and* years of parenting.

How Has What You've Learned in This Program Been Important to You?

The program has helped me learn new ways to . . .	What's your experience?
"respond to intense sensations and emotions."	
"be more aware of my experience in the present moment versus being on automatic pilot."	
"be less pulled away by worrying about the future or dwelling on the past."	
"be kinder with and less critical of myself."	
"connect with my baby."	
"relate to depression and worry thoughts (e.g., knowing that 'thoughts are not facts')."	
"accept uncertainty and difficulty as part of the path of pregnancy and parenting."	
"recognize my individual triggers and warning signs."	

From *Expecting Mindfully: Nourish Your Emotional Well-Being and Prevent Depression during Pregnancy and Postpartum,* by Sona Dimidjian and Sherryl H. Goodman. Copyright © 2019 The Guilford Press. Purchasers of this book can photocopy and/or download additional copies of this material (see the box at the end of the Contents).

It can be helpful to decide on a few options for practice—some that you can do as longer practices and some that you can integrate into the brief moments of your daily life, especially after the baby arrives.

Let's consider three categories of practice: formal practice, informal practice, and the 3-minute breathing space.

Formal Practice

Reflect on your experience this past week doing the formal practice you selected to use over the next several weeks. Would any changes to your daily practice plan be helpful? As a reminder, here is the list of formal practices:

- The body scan
- 10-minute sitting meditation
- 25-minute sitting meditation
- 10-minute yoga
- 25-minute yoga
- 10-minute walking meditation
- 20-minute lovingkindness sitting meditation
- 10-minute lovingkindness walking meditation

It is important to be realistic about what practice you select and how often and how long each practice session will be. Decide on a plan that is possible for you, rather than planning for a routine that will be hard to sustain, and thus setting yourself up for the experience of failure.

Remember that whether it is for three breaths, 3 minutes, or 30 minutes, what is important is to commit to *doing something* each day. This is even more true when parenting in the early years.

Write here what you intend for your formal practice, including both when and how long you will practice:

_____

_____

_____

_____

Informal Practice

We've practiced with many ways of bringing mindfulness into everyday life. You always can rely on the recorded instructions for "Drinking Tea Meditation" (Track 2), "Eating Meditation" (Track 3), and "Washing Dishes Meditation" (Track 4). Also, you may want to explore practicing mindfulness of other routine activities, such as the following:

- Being with your baby
- Checking e-mail or text messages
- Listening to music
- Cooking
- Waking up in the morning
- Saying good morning/good night
- Getting into bed at night
- Using the phone
- Folding laundry
- Washing dishes
- Settling into a meeting at work
- Sweeping floors
- Scrubbing tubs, floors, toilets
- Straightening up
- Taking out the garbage
- Driving
- Waiting in line
- Brushing teeth, bathing, showering
- Getting dressed
- Brushing/drying hair
- Other: _____

Parenting also offers endless opportunities for mindfulness in everyday life. In fact, after your baby is born, one of the ways you can continue to practice is by making the everyday activities of being with your baby a form of practice. Your baby can be a very valuable teacher of mindful awareness, reminding you to be present in this moment, time after time, regardless of what else you're doing. The essence of practice with your baby is bringing your attention to your direct, moment-by-moment experiences of being with your baby, and when your attention wanders, perhaps to all the many things to do as a new mom or all the worries or doubts that can arise, returning again and again to being with your baby. Here are some examples of informal practice while holding your baby:

- Allow yourself to feel the sensations of holding. As you pick up and hold your baby in your arms, know that you can take your time noticing the sensations of holding.

- Give yourself permission, for a moment, to let go of other obligations and thoughts, knowing that there is nothing to do right now other than noticing how it feels to hold your baby. Feel the weight of your baby in your arms. Where do you feel heaviness or lightness? Where does your baby make contact with your body?

- Practice with seeing your baby with openness and curiosity. Allow the sensations of touch to fade into the background, bringing your awareness to fully seeing your baby. As best you can, gaze at your baby with care and full attention. Let your eyes explore every part of your baby, examining your baby's face, head, eyes, nose, mouth, cheeks, chin, ears, etc.

The audio guides provide instruction for mindful "Being with Baby" (Track 11) and "Feeding Baby" (Track 17). We encourage you to explore both in your daily informal practice. You can do either practice for as short or long as you choose.

Finally, some women choose to use the pleasant or unpleasant events tracking as a way to bring mindfulness to everyday activities (see the end of Chapters 2 and 3 for tracking forms). Each day, notice one pleasant and one unpleasant experience, preferably while it is occurring. Record thoughts as if you were saying them out loud, in the words that actually came, and describe emotions and body sensations in as much detail as possible. Remember that the pleasant experience can be simple and brief, such as feeling the sun on your face or seeing your baby sleeping peacefully. Similarly, the unpleasant experience can be simple and brief, such as tasting an unappealing food or hearing an abrasive noise, or it can be more complicated, such as having a challenging interaction with someone. Just as a refresher, these practices also teach the skill of identifying the particular elements of an experience. Turning toward unpleasant experiences helps to provide valuable information needed to respond wisely and effectively, and noticing even small pleasant moments helps to provide nourishment.

You also might explore an audio guide that we have not used previously, "Positive Emotions" (Track 13). Because the habit of paying attention to negative and difficult experiences can be so strong, it may be helpful to build an intentional practice of paying attention to moments of pleasure. Doing so helps when we are having a rough time, allowing us to more easily remember this isn't the whole picture of who we are. Also, any time we pay attention to moments of pleasure, we give ourselves an opportunity to experience joy. In these ways, we fill up our well, which we can draw from when times are tough. We all have a capacity to pay attention to the full range of our experiences, pleasurable and difficult. Paying attention to both helps us become familiar with all of the dimensions of being pregnant, labor and delivery, and taking care of an infant. Using the guidance of Track 13, "Positive Emotions," may support you in more deeply exploring moments of happiness, joy, comfort, contentment, or gratitude.

Write here what you intend for your informal practice, including both when and how often you will practice:

_____

_____

_____

_____

The 3-Minute Breathing Space

This practice has been a great friend to many moms during pregnancy and the early parenting years, as we hope it has been for you. It's valuable as a tool for coping with challenging times—for example, a crying baby might be a reminder or signal for the coping 3-minute breathing space—and to help you pause amid all the strong emotions and thoughts that can arise when depleted and exhausted. As you know, the first step can help you step back and notice thoughts, feelings, and bodily sensations rather than getting pulled into the storm. The second and third steps can provide the ground from which you can consider which of the four doors, as described in Class 7, would be most helpful in responding to the challenge.

When the demands of caring for others are intense, the 3-minute breathing space also is valuable as your daily formal practice. You might commit to three scheduled sessions each day for the 3-minute breathing space (e.g., when you wake up, midday, and before bed).

Write here what you intend for your 3-minute breathing space practice, including both when and how often you will practice:

_____

_____

_____

_____

What Are My Potential Barriers to Practice, and How Can I Work Skillfully with Them?

Review the list that follows and check off the barriers that you anticipate may pull you off track in your daily practice.

☐ 1. I just don't have time.

☐ 2. I'm so tired.

☐ 3. I have to prioritize other people's needs over my own.

☐ 4. I feel too down or anxious to focus when I practice.

☐ 5. I have too much to do.

☐ 6. I haven't practiced for days (weeks). Why bother now?

Consider the following suggestions for ways to work skillfully with each of these barriers once you've completed this last class and continue these practices in the future.

1. I just don't have time.

Let's talk about brief practice and informal practice—these are key when formal practice is not going to be possible because of time constraints. Consider the following:

- *Identify natural windows of time in your day that you can extend for brief, formal practice.* One mom realized that she could listen to the 10-minute meditation practice in the car before driving home from work 3 days a week. Another mom didn't have time to do the 10-minute practice, so she committed to pausing for one mindful breath before she got out of the car to pick up her kids from child care.

- *Take a 3-minute breathing space.* If you don't have time for 3 minutes, take three mindful breaths. Even this can keep you connected to your mindfulness practice.

- *Pay attention to one pleasant experience.* Pay attention to the moments, even brief, when things are okay, really experiencing them.

- *Notice everyday activities.* Recall some of your most reliable informal practices. Honor the importance of these ways to practice (they are not "less than" other practices), and do them daily.

- *Make brief walking a part of your daily practice,* even mindfully walking from the living room to the kitchen. If it's been a while since you last listened to them, do a refresher practice, listening to the "Walking Meditation" or "Lovingkindness Walking Practice" instructions (Track 9 or 16). They are available to support your practice.

Know that these forms of informal practice *count*! It's important to give yourself credit for even brief informal practices. As before, we encourage you to consider what might happen if you were told that there was something you could do for a friend, and it would take only a few minutes each day. You would probably do it. Committing to some practice each day is a chance to give yourself that same kind of gift. It's not the big gestures; it's the little gestures over and over again.

2. I am so tired.

Being pregnant, having a baby, and parenting are exhausting. If you are so very tired, know you are not alone. Exhaustion might just be the most common barrier to practice for new moms and moms-to-be.

Fatigue makes everything harder. Noticing fatigue can be a cue that caring for yourself around sleep is the highest priority. One mom kept a sign on her refrigerator that said, "Fatigue makes everything worse." Mindfully noticing your energy level is a key practice, itself, in learning to care for yourself and stay well:

- *Pay attention to how your body feels.* What are the qualities of sensations in your back, shoulders, neck, eyes, etc.? Where and how do you sense fatigue and the intensity of such sensations? Knowing what you feel is the first and most important step to addressing fatigue.

- *Ask if you are "adding on" to the experience of fatigue with self-judgment.* Are you adding on thoughts like "I shouldn't be so tired" or "I should be able to handle this better"? Or are you adding on catastrophizing thoughts like "I'm never going to be able to get enough sleep"? Remember that learning to navigate pregnancy and early parenting requires just that—learning. Self-judgment and catastrophizing thoughts make it harder for everyone to learn from experience. You will have times during which you feel exhausted and depleted—that is normal; the key is continuing to learn from these experiences so that over time you are more nourished and at ease.

- *Reflect on the balance of nourishing to depleting activities over the last day or so.* Perhaps write down your activities and identify each activity as "nourishing" or "depleting," just as we did in Class 6. What do you notice in paying attention to the balance of nourishing and depleting? In what ways can you support yourself in shifting your relationship to the depleting activities or add some nourishment to help decrease your fatigue?

- *Use the four questions* (Class 7) to help you ask for support for household tasks, work, or child care.

Also, it's possible to practice even when fatigue is present. When you're too exhausted to do a 30-minute sitting practice, you have other options:

- *Explore the mindful walking practice or the yoga practice.* Some moms find that mindful movement practices are especially helpful when fatigued.

- *Experiment with the coping 3-minute breathing space when fatigue is intense.* It can be a valuable anchor in a sea of exhaustion.

- *Use the four questions* to ask for support so that you can have time to practice, even briefly—without having to wake up earlier or go to bed later at night.

3. I have to prioritize other people's needs over my own.

The demands of caring for others can make it challenging to set aside formal time for practice. A few guidelines can be helpful in working skillfully with this barrier:

- *Remind yourself that taking care of yourself helps you care for others.* It is not selfish. It is a way to be healthy. The healthier you are, the more effective you can be in caring for others.

- *Integrate your practice time with time you are caring for your baby or children.* Practice mindfulness while you're feeding your baby, walking your peaceful or fussy baby, helping your child put on shoes. When your baby is napping, place one hand on your baby's back and practice being mindful of the rhythm of your baby breathing. If you are new to practicing in this way, it can be easier to begin at a time when your baby is calm. Perhaps set aside a few minutes while your baby is sleeping—letting go of all the other things that require your attention—to do the "being with baby" practice while holding your sleeping baby. Or set aside a few minutes when your baby is feeding peacefully, using the audio Track 17 if helpful, rather than times when the baby is struggling with nursing or with the bottle or food. Practicing at such times can help you build the skill and confidence of paying attention in a kind and curious way, even during the challenging times when your baby is fussy or hard to soothe or when many responsibilities are clamoring for your attention and your own commitment to practice has been put on the back burner.

- *Include yourself and others in a circle of care by repeating the lovingkindness phrases when the demands are high*: "May we be surrounded with lovingkindness. May we treat ourselves with kindness in good times and in hard times. May we be well and live with ease."

- *Use the four questions* to ask for help or say no to other people's requests. It's a practice that gets easier with repeated use. Use it often!

4. I feel too down or anxious to focus when I practice.

If you find that depression, stress, worry, or anxiety has returned in a way that makes it hard to sustain your attention when you practice, it may be wise to reach out for extra support. You might check in with the list of warning signs that you identified in your action plan in Class 7 and review them with your support person to ask for feedback on whether your support person has noticed any of the warning signs.

Self-criticism can accompany such experiences (thoughts like "I've failed" or "What's wrong with me?"). Worry also may be present (thoughts like "I don't want depression to come back; maybe if I ignore it, it will go away"). It is important to recognize that thoughts of self-criticism or worry are parts of the territory of depression or anxiety for many.

To overcome these barriers, reach out to others:

- *Talk* with your doctor or healthcare provider. Talk with your partner or support people. It's always okay to ask for help.

- *Use the four questions* as a guide to help you reach out and ask for what will support your well-being.

5. I have too much to do.

The to-do list can be pretty powerful during pregnancy and parenting. As one mom explained, the daily tasks asserted themselves in her awareness from the earliest moments of the day: "Every day I wake up and say, 'Okay, I'm just going to go straight upstairs and do my meditating practice or yoga.' But before I do it, I find myself again thinking I can just slip in one of the endless household tasks. I'll say, 'I'm just going to throw in some laundry,' but then the laundry leads to something else, and I'm saying, 'I'll just do these dishes really quickly and then just, you know, get the bed made.' Any one of those things takes just a few minutes, but before I know it, I've done them all, and there's no time left before we have to leave, and another day goes by without my doing the practice."

Consider the following in response to the tyranny of the to-do list:

- *Ask yourself: Have you included time for "being" on your to-do list?* If it helps, take a moment to write down "being time" on your list of activities for the day.

- *Hold the long view.* Pay attention to what is wise and necessary for the future, in addition to right now. Holding the long view can help you prioritize taking care of yourself, putting "you" on your list of things to do as a priority relative to all the other people and things on your list. In the moment, the pressure for things like doing the laundry is pretty immediate: you think, "I have to do the laundry because no one has any clean underwear!" When our field of vision is narrowed to the short term, choosing the clean underwear that everyone needs right now over time for practice seems like a wise choice. Holding the long view, though, asks us to balance these immediate demands with what is wise in the long term so you can see how short-term decisions actually lead to depletion in the long term.

- *Welcome the times when you have to wait for something as opportunities to practice.* The 3-minute breathing space is a wonderful framework for practice when you're put on hold on the phone, when the line at the pharmacy or grocery store is long, when your doctor or other health care provider is running late. Or simply place a hand on your belly and notice the rise and fall with each in and out breath.

- *Notice your body as you move throughout the day, particularly in transitions.* Pay attention to the movement of your legs, your feet making contact with the ground. Where is your attention? Are you jumping into the future? Are you rushing to the next place or to the next moment, rehearsing what you will say or do when you get there or what has to get done? Bring your attention back to the moment. Feel the air on your face, the movement of your arms and legs as you walk, even hurriedly, and the contact of your feet with the ground. If you're rushing, rush mindfully.

6. I haven't practiced for days (weeks). Why bother now?

Do you set such high expectations for yourself that it's impossible to meet them and then you stop practicing altogether, rather than practicing less often or for shorter times than you had planned? Holding yourself to such high expectations may have been useful in some contexts in your life, but these perfectionistic thoughts are not likely to be a friend to you as you consider how best to integrate these practices into your life.

Similarly, "all or nothing" thinking may be part of the territory of depression that pops up, even when you're not currently depressed, telling you that all hope is lost if you haven't stayed on track.

These types of thoughts can be a major barrier to doing the practices that help you stay well. Practicing kindness, gentleness, and beginning again can be powerful antidotes. Consider the following:

- *Remember to begin again.* On the days you don't practice, the possibility of being gentle and kind with yourself and beginning again, in that very moment, is always available to you!

- *Start with something small to begin again.* Right now, take a breathing space or even just one mindful breath. Congratulate yourself for that!

- *The more that you integrate practice into the routine of your day, the easier it is to keep doing it.* In the morning when you wake up, take three mindful breaths before you get out of bed. Explore this as a morning routine or integrate it as your nighttime routine as you get into bed. Or explore being mindful while taking a shower, washing your face, or brushing your teeth as a daily practice.

- *Reach out and talk with your support person.* Talk about why this program was of value to you, reasons to begin again, and how best to respond to perfectionist or "all or nothing" thinking.

Now that you've read the suggestions, write in the form on page 194 a few possible ideas you can explore in working with potential barriers in your own practice.

Lesson 3. Sustaining a Lifetime of Practice as a Mom

Take a moment to reflect on why you originally came to this course. For example, what were your hopes? What did you want to learn?

_____

_____

_____

_____

_____

Take a moment to reflect on what kept you going with the classes and practices, even when it was challenging. For example, what were you learning? What changes did you see in your life? What was of value to you?

_____

_____

_____

_____

_____

Potential Barriers and Ways of Responding

What are my potential barriers to practice?	In what ways might I explore responding to barriers?
I just don't have time.	
I'm so tired.	
I have to prioritize other people's needs over my own.	
I feel too down or anxious to focus when I practice.	
I have too much to do.	
I haven't practiced for days (weeks). Why bother now?	

Take a moment to reflect on what matters most to you in the future and how that can be supported by sustaining a mindfulness practice. For example, what do you care about most deeply? What are your hopes and dreams for yourself and your children? What matters most to you in the near and long-term future?

_____

_____

_____

_____

_____

Looking back over what you wrote about your initial hopes and dreams, your experience of practice and learning throughout the eight classes, and your values and vision for the future, write what inspires and motivates you to keep practicing:

_____

_____

_____

_____

_____

We encourage you to explore ways to keep this intention alive and accessible to you in your everyday life. Some options include:

- *Write your inspiration on a sticky note or index card and tape it up where you'll see it every day*—bathroom mirror, refrigerator, next to your bed, above the changing table, on your computer, etc.

- *Take a picture of your written inspiration and keep it on your cell phone.* Look at it at least once a day.

- *Find a photograph or an image that symbolizes your intention*—a photo of your child, a nature scene you love, a person meditating—and hang it or post it electronically where you will see every day.

- *Pick an object that reminds you of your intention.* Some women have chosen a small heart-shaped object to symbolize the ways in which love for their children motivates them to practice. Others have chosen a stone or polished rock to symbolize the ways in which the practice helps to keep them grounded in the present moment.

One mother, at the end of her pregnancy, chose a ring that she wore every day as a reminder of her intentions to be mindful during her postpartum and early parenting years. It may be something different that works for you. What's important is that the object be connected to your intention and that it helps keep you connected to what matters most to you.

- *Put your letter to yourself, which you completed in Class 7, in a special place* that you can access and that reminds you of all that you've learned.

Congratulations!

Congratulations for completing this program! We have journeyed together through eight classes, learning and practicing. It was an honor to accompany and guide you in your learning. We encourage you to return to these chapters and audio/video guides for the practices at any point in the future. Remember that you can return to these materials again and again.

In addition, we encourage you to explore ways to engage other people to help support your practice:

- If you know of a few women (or even just one other mother) who have struggled with depression, anxiety, or stress and are open to the skills and practices that this book teaches, you might invite them to join you in meeting periodically as you return to the chapters and practices in the book.

- Invite your husband or partner to practice with you. As one mom described, "I've gotten my husband to start doing the 3-minute breathing space with me. It's good for him, and it helps me because we can remind one another about doing it when we're hitting our limit with everything going on."

- Find a local mindfulness or yoga practice group that can help to sustain and nourish your ongoing practice.

- If you are in a play group with your child, ask the other parents about integrating one mindful minute for the parents. Set a timer and a focus for your attention; for example, bring your attention to hearing the sounds of children playing for a minute, bring your attention to the feeling of your breath, or if you're outdoors, the sensations of the air on your face.

- If you're employed outside the home, explore with your coworkers ways to integrate a few moments of practice at work.

Ultimately, what matters is paying attention to the question: What will help support me on my ongoing path of well-being? We encourage you to approach this question with the same curiosity and spirit of learning that you have engaged since you started this workbook.

We wish you well.

Daily Practice Summary

We invite you to use the Practice Journal and the Circle of Support Reflections page for supporting a lifetime of practice (information on printing extra forms can be found at the end of the Contents).

Practice Journal

	What is your intention for formal and informal daily practice?	What did you experience in your practice today? What did you learn from your practice?	Did you encounter any barriers, and if so, how did you work with them?
Day 1			
Day 2			
Day 3			
Day 4			
Day 5			
Day 6			
Day 7			

From *Expecting Mindfully: Nourish Your Emotional Well-Being and Prevent Depression during Pregnancy and Postpartum,* by Sona Dimidjian and Sherryl H. Goodman. Copyright © 2019 The Guilford Press. Purchasers of this book can photocopy and/or download additional copies of this material (see the box at the end of the Contents).

Circle of Support Reflections

What is your intention for connecting with your support person this week?

What did you notice in connecting with your support person this week?

From *Expecting Mindfully: Nourish Your Emotional Well-Being and Prevent Depression during Pregnancy and Postpartum,* by Sona Dimidjian and Sherryl H. Goodman. Copyright © 2019 The Guilford Press. Purchasers of this book can photocopy and/or download additional copies of this material (see the box at the end of the Contents).

Resources

Helpful Mindfulness Resources

ACCESS MBCT

www.accessmbct.com
• ACCESS MBCT is an online, free, and searchable directory for finding MBCT therapists in your community.

Be Mindful (UK)

http://bemindful.co.uk/evidence-research
• Website sponsored by the Mental Health Foundation, which has advocated mindfulness for better mental health since 2010, offers research data on its effectiveness. Also provides links to help you find a teacher or learn mindfulness online.

Calm

www.calm.com
• Calm is a mindfulness app that features a library of guided meditations, relaxing sounds and music, short breathing exercises, and sleep stories.

Center for Mindfulness in Medicine, Health Care, and Society

www.umassmed.edu/cfm
• Information on finding (or training to become) a mindfulness-based stress reduction (MBSR) teacher, in addition to other mindfulness-based programs, including mindfulness-based cognitive therapy (MBCT).

Headspace

www.headspace.com
• Headspace is a mindfulness app that offers hundreds of themed sessions on everything from stress to sleep, bite-sized meditations for busy schedules, and SOS exercises in case of sudden meltdowns.

MBCT in Australia

www.openground.com.au/individuals/mindfulness-based-cognitive-therapy
• Connects individuals with MBCT groups in Adelaide.

MBCT in New Zealand

www.mentalhealth.org.nz/home/our-work/page/21/4/mindfulness-directory-nz
• A directory of mindfulness teachers in New Zealand.

MBCT in the United Kingdom
https://mbct.co.uk/the-mbct-programme
• Connects individuals to MBCT classes in the United Kingdom.

Mindfulness-Based Cognitive Therapy for Prevention of Depression Relapse
www.mbct.com
• Everything you need to know about MBCT from the originators of the treatment.

Mindfulness UK: Teaching, training, therapy
https://mindfulnessuk.com/mbsr
• Website for the mindfulness-based stress reduction (MBSR) program

National Health Service (UK) Choices
www.nhs.uk/conditions/stress-anxiety-depression/mindfulness
• Information on what mindfulness is, how it helps with depression and anxiety and other problems, and different mindfulness practices.

10% Happier
www.10percenthappier.com
• Offers meditation practices and teaching from leading mindfulness teachers, such as Joseph Goldstein, interviewed by best-selling author Dan Harris.

Mindfulness Resources from Sharon Salzberg

Sharon Salzberg is a leading teacher of mindfulness and compassion practices in the West. She has authored numerous books and has been leading meditation retreats around the world for decades.

www.sharonsalzberg.com/street-lovingkindness-video-series
• The *Street Lovingkindness Video Series* takes the formal meditation practice of Lovingkindness into everyday life.

www.sharonsalzberg.com/books-audio
• A list of Sharon's books.

www.sharonsalzberg.com/metta-hour-podcast
• The Metta Hour Podcast is Sharon's podcast that brings contemplative practices to everyday life in a practical, common sense way.

www.sharonsalzberg.com/on-being-column
• A column by Sharon for the public radio show and podcast "On Being"

www.sharonsalzberg.com/events
• Sharon's teaching schedule.

www.sharonsalzberg.com/resources
• Recommended meditation centers.

Resources about Depression

Anxiety and Depression Association of America
www.adaa.org
• Offers a wealth of resources for both individuals and professionals, including a therapist directory.

The Blue Dot Project
www.thebluedotproject.org
• Dedicated to raising awareness of maternal mental health disorders, proliferating the blue dot as the symbol of solidarity and support, and combating stigma and shame.

Canadian Mental Health Association
https://cmha.ca

Depression UK

http://depressionuk.org

• Depression UK is a national self-help organization helping people cope with their depression.

Mental Health America

www.nmha.org

• The United States's leading community-based nonprofit dedicated to addressing the needs of those living with mental illness and to promoting the overall mental health of all Americans through advocacy, programs, and local affiliates.

Mind

www.mind.org.uk

• A mental health charity in the United Kingdom that connects people with information and resources and strives to eliminate stigma surrounding mental health.

National Health Service (U.K.)

www.nhs.uk/conditions/post-natal-depression

• Resources on postnatal depression's symptoms and treatment.

National Institute of Mental Health

www.nimh.nih.gov/health/topics/depression/index.shtml

• Many resources on depression, from signs and symptoms of disorders to treatments and therapies, how to participate in a clinical trial, and sources of additional information.

Postpartum Support International

www.postpartum.net

• Dedicated to increasing awareness among public and professional communities about the emotional changes that women experience during pregnancy and postpartum. Disseminates information and resources through its volunteer coordinators (in each American state and 36 other countries), a website, and annual conference. Its goal is to provide current information, resources, and education, and to advocate for further research and legislation to support perinatal mental health.

Public Health Service of Canada

www.canada.ca/en/public-health/services/health-promotion/mental-health/depression-pregnancy.html

ReachOut Australia

https://au.reachout.com

• Comprehensive guide to support services for depression in Australia.

Resources for pre- and postnatal depression and anxiety in Australia

www.panda.org.au

• Offers support and referrals.

Resources for pregnant women and parenting mothers (UK)

www.nct.org.uk

2020 Mom

www.2020mom.org

• Devoted to closing gaps in maternal mental health care through education, advocacy, and collaboration. Builds nationwide partnerships with dedicated stakeholders, pursuing advocacy opportunities, providing training and tools, and promoting recommendations for hospitals, insurers and providers.

U.S. Dept. of Health and Human Services Mental Health site

www.mentalhealth.gov

• One-stop access to U.S. government mental health and mental health problems information, including information on talking about mental health, finding a peer support group, and getting help. *Mentalhealth.gov* aims to educate and guide.

Mindfulness Readings

Bays, J. C. (2014). *Mindfulness on the go: Simple meditation practices you can do anywhere.* Boston & London: Shambhala.

Brach, T. (2003). *Radical acceptance: Embracing your life with the heart of a buddha.* New York: Bantam Books.

Goldstein, J. (2013). *Mindfulness: A practical guide to awakening.* Boulder, CO: Sounds True.

Gunaratana, B. (2002). *Mindfulness in plain English.* Somerville, MA: Wisdom.

Harris, D. (2017). *Meditation for fidgety skeptics: A 10% happier how-to book.* New York: Penguin Random House.

Kabat-Zinn, J. (2012). *Mindfulness for beginners: Reclaiming the present moment—and your life.* Boulder, CO: Sounds True.

Kabat-Zinn, J., & Kabat-Zinn, M. (2010). *Everyday blessings: The inner work of mindful parenting.* New York: Hachette.

Kornfield, J. (2011). *A lamp in the darkness: Illuminating the path through difficult times.* Boulder, CO: Sounds True.

Nhat Hanh, T. (1975). *The miracle of mindfulness: An introduction to the practice of meditation.* Boston: Beacon Press.

Salzberg, S. (2011). *Real happiness: The power of meditation.* New York: Workman.

Stahl, B., & Goldstein, E. (2010). *A mindfulness-based stress reduction workbook.* Oakland, CA: New Harbinger.

Sunim, H. (2017). *The things you can see only when you slow down: How to be calm and mindful in a fast-paced world.* New York: Penguin Books.

Teasdale, J., Williams, M., & Segal, Z. (2014). *The mindful way workbook: An 8-week program to free yourself from depression and emotional distress.* New York: Guilford Press.

Williams, M., & Penman, D. (2011). *Mindfulness: An eight-week plan for finding peace in a frantic world.* New York: Rodale.

Williams, M., Teasdale, J., Segal, Z., & Kabat-Zinn, J. (2007). *The mindful way through depression.* New York: Guilford Press.

Index

Note. *f* following a page number indicates a figure.

Acceptance
  "add-on" thoughts and, 118–119
  of feelings, 33
  lovingkindness and, 136
  planning for the future and, 181–182
Action door, 163–165. *See also* "Four doors"
Action plans, 145–149, 151
Actions, warning signs and, 145–149, 151
Activities, pleasant. *See* Pleasant experiences
Activities, routine. *See* Routine activities
Acute depression, 6. *See also* Depression
"Add-on" thoughts
  overview, 113–120, 128
  Practice Journal and, 130–131
  3-minute breathing space practice and, 124–127
Allowing, 181–182
Ambiguity, 50
Anchoring in the body, 39–48. *See also* Body scan
    practice
Anchoring in the present moment, 65–66. *See also*
    Present moment awareness
Anxiety
  autopilot and, 26
  circles of connection and, 14
  preparing for a lifetime of practice, 191
  recognizing the signs of, 100–108, 109
  thoughts and, 123
  warning signs and, 133
Asking for help, 165–175
Attention
  "add-on" thoughts and, 117–119
  body scan practice and, 30–31, 34
  mindful breathing practice and, 53–55
  pleasant experiences and, 51–52
  preparing for a lifetime of practice, 186–187
  sitting meditation and, 65–66
Automatic thoughts, 50, 113–120. *See also* Thoughts

Autopilot, 26–29, 36–37, 65–66
Availability of mindfulness, 21–25. *See also*
    Mindfulness practice
Avoidance, 94
Awareness
  body scan practice and, 29–35, 40
  to daily routines, 133
  mindful awareness to everyday activities, 138–148,
    150, 152–153
  mindful movement practice and, 67
  myths about motherhood and, 156
  noticing in daily life, 73–76
  opening to difficulty and uncertainty practices, 87
  pleasant experiences and, 52, 55
  Practice Journal and, 56–57
  3-minute breathing space practice and, 77, 98

Behaviors, 145–149, 151
Being mode, 27. *See also* Autopilot
Being with baby practice
  overview, 73–76, 78–79
  points of view, 123–124
  Practice Journal and, 80–81, 110–111, 130–131
Beliefs, 155–161
Body door, 163–165. *See also* "Four doors"
Body focus. *See also* Sensations
  "add-on" thoughts and, 117–119, 128
  beginning with, 39–48
  mindful movement practice and, 67
  Practice Journal and, 56–57
  3-minute breathing space practice and, 97–99
  warning signs and, 105, 145–149, 151
Body scan practice. *See also* Mindfulness practice
  overview, 29–35, 39–48, 41–47, 55, 179–182
  Practice Journal and, 36–37, 56–57
  practicing, 47–48
  preparing for a lifetime of practice, 184

Boredom, 44
Breath
    mindful breathing practice, 53–55
    mindful stillness and movement practices, 65–66
    overview, 39, 108–109
    Practice Journal and, 56–57
    3-minute breathing space practice and, 71–73, 96–100, 109

Caring for others, 136–137, 190–191
Challenges
    asking for help and saying no and, 165–175
    barriers to practice, 188–193, 194
    body scan practice and, 42–46
    lovingkindness and, 136–137
    myths about motherhood, 155–161
    opening to difficulty and uncertainty practices, 85–96
Change, 105–108, 118
Chores, household, 191–192. See also Everyday activities
Cognitive-behavioral therapy (CBT), 2–5
Communication, 165–175
Connecting activities. See also Routine activities
    mindful awareness to everyday activities, 141–144, 150
    Practice Journal and, 152–153
    warning signs and, 147–148
Connecting with your baby, 137
Control, 94–95, 123
Critical thoughts. See also Self-criticism
    body scan practice and, 33–34
    lovingkindness and, 136, 137
    preparing for a lifetime of practice, 189, 191
Curiosity, 33, 46–47, 181–182

Daily practices. See also Mindfulness practice; Practice Journal; Reflection
    "add-on" thoughts, 119–120
    asking for help and saying no, 174–175
    autopilot, 28–29, 35
    availability of mindfulness, 26, 35
    barriers to practice, 188–193, 194
    body focus, 47–48, 55
    body scan practice, 34–35
    circles of connection and, 8
    interpretations, 51–52, 55
    lovingkindness practice, 138
    mindful awareness to everyday activities, 144–145
    mindful breathing practice, 54–55
    mindful stillness and movement practices, 70, 76
    myths about motherhood, 160–161
    noticing in daily life, 76
    opening to difficulty and uncertainty practices, 95–96
    overview, 12–16, 13f
    pleasant experiences and, 51–52

points of view, 123–124, 128
preparing for, 11–12
preparing for a lifetime of practice, 182, 184–193, 194
self-care and, 149, 150
support and, 175
thoughts and, 128
3-minute breathing space practice and, 73, 99–100, 127, 128
warning signs and, 108, 109, 148–149
Depleting activities. See also Routine activities
    asking for help and saying no and, 172–173
    mindful awareness to everyday activities, 138–145
    Practice Journal and, 152–153
    preparing for a lifetime of practice, 189–190
Depression
    in pregnant, postpartum, and early parenting women, 5–7
    preparing for a lifetime of practice, 191
    recognizing the signs of, 100–108, 109
    resources for, 202–203
    safety and, 9
    thoughts and, 123
    vulnerability to, 5–7, 50
    warning signs and, 133, 149
Difficult emotions, 45. See also Emotions
Difficulty
    "add-on" thoughts, 119–120, 128
    opening to, 85–91
    points of view, 123
    preparing for a lifetime of practice, 186–187
    recognizing the signs of depression and anxiety, 100–108
    3-minute breathing space practice and, 96–100, 128
Direct experiences, 13. See also Experiences
Discomfort, 43
Distraction during practices
    body scan practice and, 30, 34, 45
    mindfulness during pregnancy and, 78
    sitting meditation and, 65–66
Doing mode, 27. See also Autopilot
Doubts, 46
Drowsiness during practice. See Sleepiness

Early parenting
    "add-on" thoughts and, 115
    lovingkindness and, 137
    mindfulness during, 75
    myths about motherhood, 155–161
    pleasure, mastery, and connecting activities and, 141–142
    recognizing the signs of depression and anxiety, 100–108
Eating mindfully practice, 22–23, 23–25, 185
Emotions. See also Feelings
    "add-on" thoughts and, 128
    body scan practice and, 45

emotional safety and, 9
interpretations, 48–52
mindful breathing practice and, 53
opening to difficulty and uncertainty practices, 86, 92
points of view, 120–124, 128
preparing for a lifetime of practice, 186–187
thoughts and, 122–123
3-minute breathing space practice and, 97–99
warning signs and, 100–108, 105, 145–149, 151
Environment, 28–29, 44
Everyday activities. *See also* Routine activities
asking for help and saying no and, 165–166
mindful awareness to, 133, 138–145, 150
mindfulness of, 21–26
myths about motherhood and, 160–161
noticing practices and, 73–76, 78, 80–81
Practice Journal and, 36–37, 110–111, 130–131, 152–153, 175
preparing for a lifetime of practice, 185–187, 191–192
recognizing the signs of depression and anxiety, 105, 107
Exhaustion. *See* Sleepiness
Expectations, 192–193, 194
Experiences. *See also* Pleasant experiences
"add-on" thoughts and, 114–115
body scan practice and, 40
mindful awareness to everyday activities, 138–145
opening to difficulty and uncertainty practices, 89–91
3-minute breathing space practice and, 77
Exploration, 89–91

Fatigue
body scan practice and, 43, 46–47
preparing for a lifetime of practice, 189–190
working through this program and, 9–10
Feelings. *See also* Emotions
awareness to daily routines and, 133
body focus, 39–40
body scan practice and, 33
interpretations, 48–52
mindful breathing practice and, 53
opening to difficulty and uncertainty practices, 86, 93–94
points of view, 123–124, 128
Practice Journal and, 58–59, 82–83
warning signs and, 145–149, 151
Formal practice, 15, 184, 188. *See also* Daily practices; Mindfulness practice
"Four doors," 161–165, 175
Frustration, 46
Future, planning for. *See* Planning for the future

Gentleness, 46–47, 133–138
Grounding, 117–119

Help, asking for, 165–175
Household chores, 191–192. *See also* Everyday activities

Impatience, 105
Informal practice, 15, 185–187. *See also* Daily practices; Mindfulness practice
Inspiration, 195–196
Intention, 195–196
Interpersonal skills, 165–175
Interpretations, 39, 48–52, 55
Irritability, 105
Isolation, 8–9

Judgment, 26. *See also* Critical thoughts

Kindness, 133–138

Letter writing to a future self
overview, 175, 176–177
Practice Journal and, 152–153, 175
sustaining a lifetime of practice, 196
warning signs, 148–149, 150, 151
Lovingkindness practice
overview, 133–138, 149
Practice Journal and, 152–153
preparing for a lifetime of practice, 184, 189, 190–191

Mastery activities. *See also* Routine activities
mindful awareness to everyday activities, 141–144, 150
Practice Journal and, 152–153
warning signs and, 147–148
Meditation practices, 62–65. *See also* Mindfulness practice
Memories, 86
Mind wandering. *See* Wandering mind
Mindfulness practice. *See also* Body scan practice; Daily practices
"add-on" thoughts and, 114, 119–120
autopilot and, 27–28
availability of mindfulness, 21–26, 22–23
barriers to practice, 188–193, 194
breath and, 39
circles of connection and, 13–14
lovingkindness practice, 133–138
mindful breathing practice, 53–55
mindful stillness and movement practices, 62–70, 66–70
mindfulness practices, 183
myths about motherhood and, 160–161
noticing in daily life, 73–76
opening to difficulty and uncertainty practices, 85–96
overview, 2–3, 15, 196–197
planning for the future and, 179–182

Mindfulness practice (*continued*)
    preparing for a lifetime of practice, 182, 184–193, 194
    resources for, 201–202, 204
    sitting meditation and, 62–65
    sustaining a lifetime of practice, 193, 195–196
    3-minute breathing space practice and, 71–73
Mindfulness-based cognitive therapy (MBCT), 2–7
Moods, 58–59, 82–83
Motherhood, myths regarding. *See* Myths about motherhood
Movement practices. *See also* Mindfulness practice; Walking meditation; Yoga
    opening to difficulty and uncertainty practices, 95–96
    overview, 66–70, 76
    Practice Journal and, 80–81
Myths about motherhood
    asking for help and saying no, 174
    "four doors" and, 161–165
    overview, 155–161, 175
    Practice Journal and, 175

No, saying, 165–175
Noticing practices, 73–76, 78, 80–81. *See also* Everyday activities
Nourishing activities. *See also* Routine activities
    asking for help and saying no and, 172–173
    mindful awareness to everyday activities, 138–145
    Practice Journal and, 152–153
    preparing for a lifetime of practice, 189–190

Observation, 89–91
OPEN acronym
    opening to difficulty and uncertainty practices, 89–91
    overview, 95–96
    Practice Journal and, 110–111
    reflections on, 109
Openness, 85–96, 181–182

Parenting, early. *See* Early parenting
Patient Health Questionnaire–9, 105–107
Perspective, 120–124
Planning for the future. *See also* Staying-well plan
    barriers to practice, 188–193, 194
    mindfulness practices, 179–182, 183
    overview, 179
    preparing for a lifetime of practice, 182, 184–193
    sustaining a lifetime of practice, 193, 195–196
Pleasant experiences. *See also* Experiences
    "add-on" thoughts and, 114–115
    interpretations, 51–52
    mindful awareness to everyday activities, 138–145
    noticing in daily life, 75–76
    overview, 39, 55
    Practice Journal and, 56–59
    preparing for a lifetime of practice, 186–187, 188

Pleasure activities. *See also* Routine activities
    mindful awareness to everyday activities, 141–144, 150
    Practice Journal and, 152–153
    warning signs and, 147–148
Points of view, 120–124, 128
Practice Journal. *See also* Daily practices; Reflection
    "add-on" thoughts and, 119, 128
    autopilot, 28
    availability of mindfulness, 26
    body, mind, and breath and, 56–59
    difficulty and uncertainty and, 110–111
    everyday mindfulness practices and, 36–37
    mindful stillness and movement practices, 70, 80–81
    OPEN acronym and, 109
    opening to difficulty and uncertainty practices, 96
    overview, 14–15
    planning for the future and, 198
    pleasant experiences and, 51–52
    points of view, 124
    self-care and, 152–153
    support and, 176–177
    thoughts and, 130–131
    3-minute breathing space practice and, 73
    unpleasant experiences and, 82–83
Practices, daily. *See* Daily practices
Pregnancy
    "add-on" thoughts and, 115
    mindfulness during, 74, 78–79
    myths about motherhood, 155–161
    pleasure, mastery, and connecting activities and, 141–142
    recognizing the signs of depression and anxiety, 100–108
Present moment awareness
    "add-on" thoughts and, 114–115, 117–119
    body scan practice and, 34
    mindful stillness and movement practices, 65–66
    opening to difficulty and uncertainty practices, 89–91
    sustaining a lifetime of practice, 195–196
Pushing away, 94

Questioning
    "add-on" thoughts and, 125
    asking for help and saying no and, 166–169, 172–174, 190, 191
    Practice Journal and, 130–131

Reaction, 89–91
Reentry door, 162–165. *See also* "Four doors"
Reflection. *See also* Daily practices; Practice Journal
    "add-on" thoughts and, 116–117, 126–127
    availability of mindfulness, 23–25
    body focus, 41–47
    body scan practice, 31–35
    everyday mindfulness practices and, 35
    "four doors" and, 164–165

lovingkindness practice, 134–136

mindful stillness and movement practices, 63–65, 68–70

mindfulness practices, 180–181, 183

opening to difficulty and uncertainty practices, 87–89, 92–95

overview, 13–14, 13*f*

planning for the future and, 179, 198

thoughts and, 128

3-minute breathing space practice and, 71–72, 97–99, 126–127

Relapse prevention, 14, 100–108. *See also* Planning for the future; Staying-well plan

Relaxation, 45, 88

Responding to difficulty, 86–87, 89–91, 91–92. *See also* Difficulty

Rhythms, 61–62, 73–76, 105

Risk factors for depression during pregnancy, postpartum, and early parenting, 5–7, 28, 50. *See also* Depression

Routine activities. *See also* Everyday activities; Staying-well plan

interpretations, 52

mindful awareness to, 133, 138–145, 150

myths about motherhood and, 160–161

noticing in daily life, 73–76

pleasure, mastery, and connecting activities and, 141–144

points of view, 123–124, 128

Practice Journal and, 110–111, 130–131, 152–153

preparing for a lifetime of practice, 185–187, 189–190, 191–192

3-minute breathing space practice and, 73

warning signs and, 105, 107, 109, 147–148

Saying no, 165–175

Self-care. *See also* Planning for the future; Staying-well plan

asking for help and saying no and, 165–175

letter writing to a future self, 148, 151

lovingkindness practice, 133–138

mindful awareness to everyday activities, 138–145

overview, 133

Practice Journal and, 152–153

preparing for a lifetime of practice, 184–193, 194

warning signs, 145–149, 151

Self-criticism. *See also* Critical thoughts

autopilot and, 26

body scan practice and, 33–34, 44–45

preparing for a lifetime of practice, 189, 191

Self-doubt, 44–45

Self-judgment, 189. *See also* Self-criticism

Self-support, 18–19. *See also* Support

Sensations. *See also* Body focus

"add-on" thoughts and, 117–119, 128

body scan practice and, 33

opening to difficulty and uncertainty practices, 86, 93–94

recognizing the signs of depression and anxiety, 107–108

3-minute breathing space practice and, 97–99

Sensory experiences

autopilot and, 27–28

availability of mindfulness, 21–25

mindfulness during pregnancy and, 78–79

Practice Journal and, 58–59, 82–83

Sitting meditation

breath and, 65–66

opening to difficulty and uncertainty practices, 87, 95–96

overview, 62–65, 70, 76, 108–109

preparing for a lifetime of practice, 184

Sleepiness

body scan practice and, 43, 46–47

preparing for a lifetime of practice, 189–190

working through this program and, 9–10

Staying-well plan. *See also* Planning for the future; Self-care

asking for help and saying no and, 165–175

body scan practice and, 42

mindful awareness to everyday activities, 144

mindful stillness and movement practices, 64

opening to difficulty and uncertainty practices, 95

overview, 179

recognizing the signs of depression and anxiety, 100–108

reflections on, 24–25

Stillness, mindful

overview, 76, 108–109

Practice Journal and, 80–81

sitting meditation and, 62–66, 70, 76

Stress, 100, 133

Support. *See also* Self-support

asking for help and saying no and, 165–175

circles of connection and, 8–9

difficulty and uncertainty and, 109

identifying a support person, 15–19

inviting and sustaining, 16–19

myths about motherhood, 155–161

overview, 155

preparing for a lifetime of practice, 191

recognizing the signs of depression and anxiety, 109

rhythms and, 78–79

thoughts and, 128

Symptoms. *See also* Warning signs

circles of connection and, 14

letter writing to a future self, 148, 151

overview, 5–7, 107

Thought door, 163–165. *See also* "Four doors"

Thoughts

"add-on" thoughts and, 113–120, 128

body focus, 39–40

interpretations, 48–52

mindful breathing practice and, 53

Thoughts (*continued*)
  mindful stillness and movement practices, 64, 65–66
  mindfulness and, 22
  myths about motherhood and, 155–161
  opening to difficulty and uncertainty practices, 86, 93–94
  points of view, 120–124, 128
  Practice Journal and, 58–59, 82–83, 130–131
  recognizing the signs of depression and anxiety, 100–108, 105
  sitting meditation and, 65–66
  warning signs and, 145–149, 151
3-minute breathing space practice
  "four doors" and, 161–165
  overview, 71–73, 77, 96–100, 109, 124–127, 128, 155, 175
  Practice Journal and, 80–81, 110–111, 130–131, 175
  preparing for a lifetime of practice, 187, 188, 192
  warning signs and, 148
Time investment
  body scan practice and, 46
  preparing for a lifetime of practice, 188–189, 191–192
  working through this program and, 9–10
Tiredness
  body scan practice and, 43, 46–47
  preparing for a lifetime of practice, 189–190
  working through this program and, 9–10
To-do lists, 191–192
Truth, 114, 119, 123

Uncertainty
  opening to, 91–96
  points of view, 123
  recognizing the signs of depression and anxiety, 100–108
  3-minute breathing space practice and, 96–100

Unpleasant events. *See also* Routine activities
  noticing in daily life, 75–76
  Practice Journal and, 82–83
  preparing for a lifetime of practice, 186–187

Vulnerability to depression, 5–7, 28, 50. *See also* Depression

Walking meditation
  opening to difficulty and uncertainty practices, 95–96
  overview, 68, 70
  preparing for a lifetime of practice, 184, 188–189, 194
Wandering mind
  body scan practice and, 30, 34, 45
  mindfulness during pregnancy and, 78
  sitting meditation and, 65–66
Warning signs. *See also* Symptoms
  asking for help and saying no, 175
  letter writing to a future self, 148, 151
  overview, 133, 145–149, 150, 151
  Practice Journal and, 152–153
  preparing for a lifetime of practice, 191
  recognizing, 5–7, 100–108, 109
Wellness. *See* Staying-well plan
Worry. *See also* Anxiety
  autopilot and, 26
  recognizing the signs of depression and anxiety, 102–104, 109
  thoughts and, 123

Yoga
  opening to difficulty and uncertainty practices, 87–88, 96
  overview, 67–68, 70, 109
  preparing for a lifetime of practice, 184

About the Authors

Sona Dimidjian, PhD, is Professor in the Department of Psychology and Neuroscience at the University of Colorado Boulder. She is a leading expert on the science and practice of promoting mental health and wellness among women, children, and families, including during pregnancy and early parenting.

Sherryl H. Goodman, PhD, is Samuel Candler Dobbs Professor of Psychology at Emory University. A widely recognized authority on mothers who have experienced depression, and their children, she also develops and tests evidence-based ways to prevent and treat depression in mothers.

List of Audio and Video Tracks

Audio Tracks

1. Introduction to Daily Activities
2. Drinking Tea Meditation
3. Eating Meditation
4. Washing Dishes Meditation
5. The Body Scan
6. Introduction to Sitting
7. 10-Minute Breathing Meditation
8. 25-Minute Sitting Meditation
9. Walking Meditation
10. 3-Minute Breathing Space
11. Being with Baby
12. Difficult Emotions
13. Positive Emotions
14. Lovingkindness Meditation Introduction
15. 20-Minute Lovingkindness Meditation Sitting Practice
16. 10-Minute Lovingkindness Walking Practice
17. Feeding Baby

Video Tracks

1. Yoga Introduction
2. 10-Minute Yoga Practice
3. 25-Minute Yoga Practice

The tracks are available to download or stream from The Guilford Press website at *www.guilford.com/dimidjian-materials*.

Terms of Use

The publisher grants to individual purchasers of *Expecting Mindfully* nonassignable permission to stream and download the audio and video files located at *www.guilford.com/dimidjian-materials*. This license is limited to you, the individual purchaser, for personal use. This license does not grant the right to reproduce these materials for resale, redistribution, broadcast, or any other purposes (including but not limited to books, pamphlets, articles, video- or audiotapes, blogs, file-sharing sites, Internet or intranet sites, and handouts or slides for lectures, workshops, or webinars, whether or not a fee is charged) in audio form or in transcription. Permission to reproduce these materials for these and any other purposes must be obtained in writing from the Permissions Department of Guilford Publications.